MOISTURIZERS

AF061322

MOISTURIZERS

Editor

Rashmi Sarkar MD MNAMS
Professor
Department of Dermatology
Maulana Azad Medical College and
Associated LNJP Hospital
New Delhi, India

Assistant Editor

Shilpa Garg MBBS DNB
Consultant
Department of Dermatology
Sir Ganga Ram Hospital
New Delhi, India

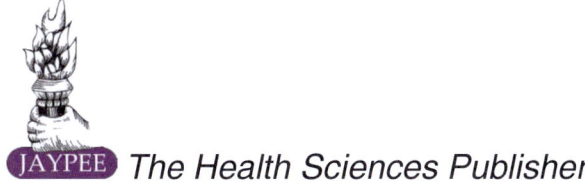

The Health Sciences Publisher
New Delhi | London | Philadelphia | Panama

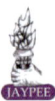 **Jaypee Brothers Medical Publishers (P) Ltd**

Headquarters

Jaypee Brothers Medical Publishers (P) Ltd
4838/24, Ansari Road, Daryaganj
New Delhi 110 002, India
Phone: +91-11-43574357
Fax: +91-11-43574314
Email: jaypee@jaypeebrothers.com

Overseas Offices

J.P. Medical Ltd
83 Victoria Street, London
SW1H 0HW (UK)
Phone: +44 20 3170 8910
Fax: +44 (0)20 3008 6180
Email: info@jpmedpub.com

Jaypee Medical Inc
325 Chestnut Street
Suite 412, Philadelphia, PA 19106, USA
Phone: +1 267-519-9789
Email: support@jpmedus.com

Jaypee Brothers Medical Publishers (P) Ltd
Bhotahity, Kathmandu, Nepal
Phone: +977-9741283608
Email: kathmandu@jaypeebrothers.com

Jaypee-Highlights Medical Publishers Inc
City of Knowledge, Bld. 235, 2nd Floor, Clayton
Panama City, Panama
Phone: +1 507-301-0496
Fax: +1 507-301-0499
Email: cservice@jphmedical.com

Jaypee Brothers Medical Publishers (P) Ltd
17/1-B Babar Road, Block-B, Shaymali
Mohammadpur, Dhaka-1207
Bangladesh
Mobile: +08801912003485
Email: jaypeedhaka@gmail.com

Website: www.jaypeebrothers.com
Website: www.jaypeedigital.com

© 2017, Jaypee Brothers Medical Publishers

The views and opinions expressed in this book are solely those of the original contributor(s)/author(s) and do not necessarily represent those of editor(s) of the book.

All rights reserved. No part of this publication may be reproduced, stored or transmitted in any form or by any means, electronic, mechanical, photocopying, recording or otherwise, without the prior permission in writing of the publishers.

All brand names and product names used in this book are trade names, service marks, trademarks or registered trademarks of their respective owners. The publisher is not associated with any product or vendor mentioned in this book.

Medical knowledge and practice change constantly. This book is designed to provide accurate, authoritative information about the subject matter in question. However, readers are advised to check the most current information available on procedures included and check information from the manufacturer of each product to be administered, to verify the recommended dose, formula, method and duration of administration, adverse effects and contraindications. It is the responsibility of the practitioner to take all appropriate safety precautions. Neither the publisher nor the author(s)/editor(s) assume any liability for any injury and/or damage to persons or property arising from or related to use of material in this book.

This book is sold on the understanding that the publisher is not engaged in providing professional medical services. If such advice or services are required, the services of a competent medical professional should be sought.

Every effort has been made where necessary to contact holders of copyright to obtain permission to reproduce copyright material. If any have been inadvertently overlooked, the publisher will be pleased to make the necessary arrangements at the first opportunity.

Inquiries for bulk sales may be solicited at: jaypee@jaypeebrothers.com

Moisturizers / Rashmi Sarkar

First Edition: **2017**

ISBN: 978-93-5250-011-6

Printed at

Dedicated to

My family and all my colleagues who believe in rational science.

Contents

Contributors ix
Preface xi

1. **Classification and Basics of Moisturizers** 1
   Shilpa Garg, Rashmi Sarkar

2. **Myths and Misconceptions About Moisturizers** 7
   Latika Arya

3. **Skin Barrier, Stratum Corneum Maturation and Moisturization** 11
   Aayushi Mehta, Rashmi Sarkar

4. **Indications of Moisturizers in Skin** 16
   Pooja Arora

5. **Moisturizers in Atopic Dermatitis** 23
   Sumit Sethi

6. **Moisturizers in Acne** 29
   Rashmi Sarkar, Shilpa Garg

7. **Moisturizers in Rosacea and Sensitive Skin** 37
   Surabhi Sinha

8. **Moisturizers for Xerotic and Ichthyotic Skin** 45
   Sayantani Chakraborty, Joyeeta Chowdhury

9. **Maintaining Skin Integrity and Moisturizers in Aged** 54
   Sidharth Sonthalia

10. **Steroid-Sparing Emollients in Dermatology** 62
    Koushik Lahiri, Abhijit Saha, Shilpa Garg

11. **Neonatal and Infantile Skin Care and Moisturizers** 69
    Indrashis Podder, Rashmi Sarkar

12. **Moisturizers and Barrier Creams in Hand Eczema** 73
    Rahul Arora, Pallavi Ailawadi

13. **Moisturizing Different Racial Skin Types** 82
    Michelle Rodrigues

14.	Moisturizers for Indian Skin: Geographical, Cultural and Regional Variations *Ishad Aggarwal, Sahil Mrigpuri*	89
15.	Natural Emollients *Narendra Gokhale*	95
16.	Use of Moisturizers in Conditions of Hyperpigmentation *Seemal R Desai, Abhijeet K Jha, Rashmi Sarkar*	100
17.	Adverse Effects of Moisturizers *Priyanka Borde Bisht, Shilpa Garg*	104
18.	Moisturizers for Hair and Nails *Soumya Jagadeesan*	108
19.	Recent Update on Moisturizers *Anupam Das, Rashmi Sarkar*	114
	Appendix	*119*

Contributors

Editor

Rashmi Sarkar MD MNAMS
Professor, Department of Dermatology
Maulana Azad Medical College and Associated LNJP Hospital
New Delhi, India

Assistant Editor

Shilpa Garg MBBS DNB
Consultant, Department of Dermatology
Sir Ganga Ram Hospital
New Delhi, India

Contributing Authors

Ishad Aggarwal MD
Senior Resident
Department of Dermatology
Institute of Post Graduate Medical Education and Research
Kolkata, West Bengal, India

Pallavi Ailawadi MD
Consultant
Department of Dermatology
Kaya Skin Clinic
New Delhi, India

Pooja Arora MBBS MD DNB MNAMS
Assistant Professor
Department of Dermatology
Post Graduate Institute of Medical Education and Research and
Dr RML Hospital
New Delhi, India

Rahul Arora MD
Senior Resident
Department of Dermatology and STD
University College of Medical Sciences and Guru Teg Bahadur Hospital
New Delhi, India

Latika Arya MBBS MD
Consultant
LA Skin and Aesthetic Clinic
New Delhi, India

Priyanka Borde Bisht MBBS DNB
Consultant, The Apollo Clinic
Pune, Maharashtra, India

Sayantani Chakraborty MD
RMO Cum Clinical Tutor
Department of Dermatology
NRS Medical College and Hospital
Kolkata, West Bengal, India

Joyeeta Chowdhury MD
RMO cum Clinical Tutor
Department of Dermatology
NRS Medical College and Hospital
Kolkata, West Bengal, India

Anupam Das MD
Senior Resident
Department of Dermatology
KPC Medical College and Hospital
Kolkata, West Bengal, India

Seemal R Desai MD FAAD
Clinical Assistant Professor
Department of Dermatology
University of Texas Southwestern Medical Center
Founder and Medical Director
Innovative Dermatology
Dallas, Texas, USA

Narendra Gokhale MBBS MD
Consultant, Sklinic
Indore, Madhya Pradesh, India

Soumya Jagadeesan MD
Assistant Professor
Department of Dermatology
Amrita Institute of Medical Sciences
Kochi, Kerala, India

Abhijeet K Jha MD
Senior Resident
Department of Dermatology, STD and Leprosy
All India Institute of Medical Sciences
Patna, Bihar, India

Koushik Lahiri MBBS DVD FAAD FFAADV FIAD MRCPS FRCP
Senior Consultant Dermatologist
Apollo Gleneagles Hospitals and WIZDERM
Kolkata, West Bengal, India

Aayushi B Mehta MBBS
Resident
Department of Dermatology
DY Patil University School of Medicine
Mumbai, Maharashtra, India

Sahil Mrigpuri MBBS MD
Junior Resident
Department of Dermatology
Post Graduate Institute of Medical Education and Research
Chandigarh, Punjab, India

Indrashis Podder MBBS
Resident
Department of Dermatology
Medical College and Hospital
Kolkata, West Bengal, India

Michelle Rodrigues MBBS FACD
Consultant
Department of Dermatology
St Vincent's Hospital
The Royal Children's Hospital
Melbourne, Australia

Abhijit Saha MBBS MD
Consultant Dermatologist
Rita Skin Foundation
Kolkata, West Bengal, India

Sumit Sethi MBBS MD DNB
Consultant Dermatologist
Dr Sethi's Genesis Skin Clinic
Genesis Hospital
New Delhi, India

Surabhi Sinha MBBS MD DNB MNAMS
Specialist
Department of Dermatology, STD and Leprosy
Dr RML Hospital, PGIMER
New Delhi, India

Sidharth Sonthalia MBBS MD DNB MNAMS FISD
Medical Director and Senior Consultant
Skinnocence: The Skin Clinic and Research Centre
Gurgaon, Haryana, India

Preface

We all use moisturizers in our daily life, but interestingly there are hardly any books on the science and art of moisturizers. When I decided to edit this book, I realized that there are many aspects of moisturizers and its uses in dermatology. Along with a group of authors, we embarked on a journey to provide facts and enjoyable reading.

I would like to thank the Assistant Editor, Dr Shilpa Garg for working diligently with me and being wonderfully receptive. A special word of thanks to Dr Neeraj Chowdhury, Senior Acquisition Editor/Corporate from Jaypee Brothers Publications with whom I worked closely and Ms Hansika Seth in the final stages. My son, Abhik S Basu, always boosts up my morale and this book would not have been possible without him, or the rest of my family who supported me especially my sister, Dr Urmi Sarkar, who gave many important scientific inputs. I am grateful to the unflinching support of my authors who worked with me inspite of a busy practice, a special mention of Drs Narendra Gokhale, Latika Arya, and Sidharth Sonthalia must be made. I also thank the almighty for giving me the strength to complete this book in my hectic schedule.

Rashmi Sarkar

CHAPTER 1

Classification and Basics of Moisturizers

Shilpa Garg, Rashmi Sarkar

INTRODUCTION

Moisturizers are formulations which help in maintaining 10–30% water content of the skin. Moisturizers constitute the most prevalent and the most important component of all skin care products. Moisturizers have a critical role in daily maintenance of healthy skin and in the treatment of certain dermatoses. By replacing the natural skin oils, covering tiny fissures and providing a protective film on the skin, moisturizers help to decrease the evaporation of the skin's moisture, maintain hydration and improve the appearance and tactile properties of skin.[1] Stratum corneum plays a key role in the development of skin barrier that has the ability to retain moisture and protects underlying tissues from infection, desiccation, chemical and mechanical stress. However, some normal movement of water takes place through the stratum corneum into the surrounding atmosphere, called as transepidermal water loss (TEWL). In patients with healthy skin with intact skin barrier TEWL is low. It is significantly high in diseases like atopic dermatitis, eczema and psoriasis. Transepidermal water loss assess the efficacy of moisturizers by its ability to reduce TEWL. Terms like emolliency, moisturizing and lubrication are often used interchangeably. Emolliency is the ability of the product to fill the crevices present between the desquamating corneocytes. Moisturizing is the net decrease in TEWL after application of the product. Lubrication is the ability of the product to improve the smoothness of skin.[1] In essence, moisturizers mimic the role of skin lipids to decrease TEWL and increase water content of the skin in order to regain and maintain an intact skin barrier. Stratum corneum is hydrated by upward movement of water from the deeper epidermal layers to stratum corneum which eventually gets lost to evaporation. Water loss through normal healthy skin occurs through sweating and TEWL.

CLASSIFICATION OF MOISTURIZERS

Moisturizers can be classified broadly into four classes: (1) occlusive, (2) humectant, (3) emollient, and (4) rejuvenator (Table 1).

Table 1: Classification of moisturizers

Classification	Mechanism of action	Advantages	Disadvantages	Prototype
Occlusives	Forms hydrophobic layer on skin surface, prevents evaporation and provides an exogenous barrier to water loss	Can significantly reduce trans-epidermal water loss and hence are most effective moisturizers; well tolerated	Greasy, allergic contact dermatitis (lanolin), comedogenic, folliculitis (mineral oil)	Petrolatum Dimethicone
Humectants	Enhances absorption of water from the dermis into the epidermis	–	Humectants have to be combined with occlusives in formulations because if used alone they can cause excessive water loss from the dermis through evaporation into the environment. Urea and lactic acid can cause irritation	Glycerin
Emollients	Fill the gaps between the corneocytes	Improves the texture and appearance of skin making it soft and smooth with improvement in overall appearance	–	Essential fatty acids like linoleic acid, cholesterol, squalene
Rejuvenators	Replenish essential proteins in the skin	–	Relatively large size of these proteins may hinder their penetration in the stratum corneum	

Occlusive

Occlusives are the most common type of moisturizers used in formulations and works by forming a hydrophobic layer on skin surface, allowing upward percolation of water from the viable epidermis but preventing evaporation through skin and providing a physical barrier to TEWL. Their effectivity can be increased by application on dampened skin as they prevent evaporation from the skin surface. For restoring skin barrier, semipermeable dressings are more desirable than complete occlusive dressings as complete occlusion does not initiate lipid synthesis due to reduction of the TEWL to zero. Occlusive ingredients include petrolatum, mineral oil, dimethicone and caprylic/capric triglyceride.

Petrolatum is prototypic of this group and is the most effective moisturizer. Petrolatum jelly in a concentration of 5% can reduce the TEWL by 99% whereas other oils decrease TEWL by only 20–30%. The ability of petroleum jelly to diffuse into the intercellular lipid domains also contributes to its efficacy. Though well tolerated, they are not very appealing due to their greasy feel. After water, petrolatum is the most commonly used active agent in the skin care products. Occlusives are used in the treatment of atopic dermatitis. A study found both an over-the-counter petroleum-based skin moisturizer and an expensive ceramide-containing prescription barrier cream to be equally effective in the treatment of mild-to-moderate atopic dermatitis.[2] Petrolatum can penetrate into the upper layers of the stratum corneum and initiate the production of intercellular lipids such as free sterols, sphingolipids and free fatty acids which help in restoring the stratum corneum barrier. Petrolatum can also reduce the appearance of fine lines caused due to dehydration.

Dimethicone is the second most commonly used active agent in moisturizers due to its hypoallergenic, noncomedogenic, nonacnegenic properties and because it does not have a strong odor. It belongs to the family of silicones which forms the basis of all oil-free preparations of moisturizers.

As compared to dimethicone, petrolatum is considered superior for skin healing and for decreasing the fine facial lines caused by dehydration. Dimethicone being permeable to water vapor cannot reduce TEWL in skin with compromised barrier. However this property is useful in formulating foundations and sunscreens as it allows for evaporation of perspiration and prevents the skin from feeling warm.

Apart from the occlusive properties, both petrolatum and dimethicone have emollient properties and can fill the spaces between the desquamating corneocytes, leading to smooth and soft skin. Lanolin is expensive, has a characteristic odor and can cause allergic contact dermatitis. Therefore, it is rarely used in moisturizers (Table 2).

Humectant

Humectants work by enhancing the absorption of water from the dermis into the epidermis. There is some evidence that humectants may also hydrate stratum corneum by absorbing water from the external environment.[3] Unlike occlusives, humectants possess hydrophilic hydroxyl groups whose hydroscopic properties

Table 2: Categories of occlusive moisturizer

Categories	Examples
Hydrocarbon oils and waxes	Petrolatum, paraffin, squalene, mineral oil
Vegetable and animal oil	Cocoa butter, lanolin
Fatty acids	Lanolin acids and stearic acid
Fatty alcohol	Lanolin alcohol, cetyl alcohol
Polyhydric alcohol	Propylene glycol
Wax esters	Lanolin, beeswax, stearyl stearate
Vegetable waxes	Carnauba, candelilla
Phospholipids	Lecithin
Sterols	Cholesterol
Silicones	Dimethicone, cyclomethicone

helps to attract and hold water molecules. Humectants are always combined with occlusives in formulations because if used alone they can cause excessive water loss from the dermis through evaporation into the environment with lower humidity, especially in those with compromised skin barrier. Humectants include glycerin, urea, sorbitol, sodium lactate, ammonium lactate, propylene glycol, sodium pyrrolidone carboxylic acid, gelatin, potassium lactate, hyaluronic acid, vitamins and proteins, and alpha hydroxyl acids like lactic acid. Glycerol or glycerin is the prototype of this group and is most effective humectant. Apart from hydroscopic properties, glycerin can also activate transglutaminase activity leading to accelerated maturation of corneocytes and reduced scaling in xerotic skin.[3] By modulating the aquaporin water channels in the epidermis, the moisturizing effect of glycerin lasts even when it is no longer present in the skin. Glycerin prevents humidity-induced crystal phase transitions in the lipids of the stratum corneum and hence improves the barrier function of the skin.[4] Glycerin may also possess corneodesmolytic properties which aids in the proteolytic degradation of corneodesmosomes, leading to desquamation. The performance of moisturizing formulations can be dramatically changed by changing the amount of humectants (especially glycerin) in a formulation. Urea has humectant properties in concentrations of up to 10%, but in higher concentrations of 20–30% it behaves like a mild keratolytic agent.

Emollient

Emollients are oils and lipids that improve the texture and appearance of the skin by filling the gaps between the corneocytes, improving the lubricity, and restoring the epidermal lipids making the skin soft, supple, flexible and smooth with improvement in overall appearance. Emollients include essential fatty acids which are present in various natural oils. Some of these essential fatty acids like linoleic acid can influence the skin physiology as they can be oxidized to eicosanoids which are important signaling molecules in the inflammatory pathways and immune system.[3] Other emollient ingredients include alcohol and alcohol esters such as octyl dodecanol, hexyl decanol, oleyl alcohol, oleyl oleate, octyl stearate, polyethylene glycol (PEG)-7 glyceryl cocoate, glycol stearate, glyceryl stearate, soy sterol, coco caprylate/caprate, myristyl myristate, cetearyl isononanoate, isopropyl myristate, etc. Based on the characteristics of greasiness and spreadability, emollients can be categorized into:[5]

1. Poor spreading/greasy emollients like castor oil, almond oil and oleyl oleate.
2. Medium spreading/creamy emollients like caprylic/capric triglyceride, octyl dodecanol, cetearyl isononanoate and oleyl alcohol.
3. Easy spreading/nongreasy emollients like dioctyl cyclohexane, isopropyl stearate and isopropyl myristate.

Rejuvenator

Rejuvenators like collagen, keratin and elastin help in replenishing the essential proteins in the skin. The relatively large size of these proteins may hinder their penetration in the stratum corneum.[6] They can also act as emollients and improve the esthetic appearance of the skin by making it smooth and stretching it to fill the fine lines. Protein additives may fill the irregularities in the stratum corneum and may provide temporary relief for dry skin. Upon drying they shrink slightly, leaving a protein film that smoothens the skin and stretch out the fine lines.

Ceramide

Ceramides are not regarded as a class of moisturizer, but are included as these lipid molecules are being increasingly used in the treatment of atopic dermatitis and in cosmeceuticals. Ceramides are present in the stratum corneum and maintain the integrity of the skin barrier. Their levels are greatly reduced in patients with atopic dry skin. Ceramides are present in many moisturizers used for treating both atopic and normal skin. Oil solubility of ceramides helps in their easy incorporation into moisturizers. However, preparations containing ceramides are very expensive.

Combination Approach

Most of the moisturizing formulations contain a combination of emollients (lipids) and humectants (glycerin) as it increases the ability of glycerin to supplement the natural moisturizing factor moisturizing system as lipid-based moisturization is disturbed in dry skin as well. There is evidence that lipids are more effective when formulated with glycerin.[4]

Prescription Device Moisturizers

Moisturizers have long been available as an over-the-counter product, however several prescription moisturizers have been recently introduced which are classified as medical devices (and not drugs) and approved by the Food and Drug Administration. Recent studies have shown equivalence of these prescription devices to less expensive over-the-counter moisturizers in the treatment of diseases such as eczema and atopic dermatitis.[6]

CHALLENGES AND LIMITATIONS IN ASSESSMENT

There are certain limitations in the mechanisms involving the evaluation of a moisturizer. The various techniques which are used to evaluate the efficacy of moisturizers are:[7]
- Skin barrier function assessed by TEWL
- Skin hydration assessed by skin hygrometers (electrical; e.g., capacitance and conductance) or spectroscopy (e.g., acoustic, infrared and nuclear magnetic resonance)
- Visual assessment by photography, videomicroscopy, expert visual grading or subject self-assessment
- Skin elasticity assessed by various biomechanical techniques (e.g., ballistometer and dermal torque meter) or by pinch recoil.

Transepidermal water loss, which is most commonly used to measure the efficacy of moisturizer, has many limitations and drawbacks. It can be influenced by humidity, stress, temperature and circadian rhythms. The devices which are used to measure TEWL may also suffer from shortcomings. Some studies have shown no correlation between the measured TEWL and skin barrier function.[8]

MARKET FORMULATIONS

Moisturizers are generally marketed in two categories: face care (with specialized products for lips and eyes) and hand and body care (with specialized products for hand and nail, and feet). Moisturizers designed for the face are nongreasy, noncomedogenic, with an emphasis on skin feel and esthetics. Silicone derivatives, kaolin and talc are added to absorb oil and reduce the facial shine. Hand and body care moisturizers mainly target prevention and treatment of dry skin. Some specialized products may include the reduction of cellulite, firming agents, bronzing, and minimizing the signs of aging.[9] Moisturizers with antiaging technology are the fastest growing segment of facial moisturizer. Sun protectants, alpha hydroxy acids (e.g., glycolic acid), ascorbic acid, retinol and its derivatives possess antiaging properties and are the special ingredients which are added to moisturizers.

CONCLUSION

Moisturizers mimic the physiological mechanism of the skin and preserve skin barrier, enhance the water-holding capacity and influence the esthetic properties of the skin. The industry for moisturizers is enormous. Majority of the products contain fundamental ingredients like glycerin, dimethicone and petrolatum, which can improve the integrity of the skin barrier, reduce fine lines, and make skin appear smooth and soft. Newer formulations containing ceramides and prescription-device moisturizers are increasingly becoming common. Moisturizers have various beneficial effects on the skin. Their effectivity will be judged by utilizing histologic, gene and protein expression in future studies.

REFERENCES

1. Lipozenčić J, Pastar Z, Marinović-Kulišić S. Moisturizers. Acta Dermatovenerol Croat 2006;14(2):104-8.
2. Miller DW, Koch SB, Yentzer BA, et al. An over-the-counter moisturizer is as clinically effective as, and more costeffective than, prescription barrier creams in the treatment of children with mild to moderate atopic dermatitis: a randomized, controlled trial. J Drugs Dermatol. 2011;10(5):531-7.
3. Anderson PC, Dinulos JG. Are the new moisturizers more effective? Curr Opin Pediatr. 2009;21(4):486-90.
4. Rawlings AV, Canestrari DA, Dobkowski B. Moisturizer technology versus clinical performance. Dermatol Ther. 2004;17 Suppl 1:49-56.
5. Draelos ZD. Therapeutic moisturizers. Dermatol Clin. 2000;18(4):597-607.
6. Nolan K, Marmur E. Moisturizers: reality and the skin benefits. Dermatol Ther. 2012;25(3):229-33.
7. Lynde C. Moisturizers for the treatment of inflammatory skin conditions. J Drugs Dermatol. 2008;7(11):1038-43.
8. Chilcott RP, Jenner J, Hotchkiss SA, et al. Evaluation of barrier creams against sulphur mustard. I. In vitro studies using human skin. Skin Pharmacol Appl Skin Physiol. 2002;15(4):225-35.
9. Kraft JN, Lynde CW. Moisturizers: what they are and a practical approach to product selection. Skin Therapy Lett. 2005;10(5):1-8.

CHAPTER 2

Myths and Misconceptions About Moisturizers

Latika Arya

INTRODUCTION

Moisturizers are very commonly prescribed in dermatological practice. Moisturizer is a generic term which encompasses a variety of formulations employed for repair of skin barrier, reduce transepidermal water loss, or esthetic improvement of dry skin.[1]

Their use may be just a part of routine skin care regimen or may be used therapeutically for various dry skin conditions like xerosis, ichthyosis, atopic dermatitis, psoriasis, etc. Although the causes, symptoms, and severity of dry skin vary widely, moisturizers form the mainstay of treatment in simple cases and can be used as adjunctive therapy in more serious clinical cases. However, there are many myths and misconceptions about moisturizers regarding their type, use and ingredients.

This chapter aims to clarify some common prevailing myths and misconceptions about moisturizers in the dermatology community (Box 1).

Myth: Oily skin does not need moisturizing.
Truth: While there is no doubt that oiliness of the skin should be controlled to prevent acne, however oily skin too needs hydration. Completely drying out oily skin sends a signal to the sebaceous glands to produce even more oil. However, the right kind of moisturizer should be chosen for oily skin.

Myth: All moisturizers are essentially the same.
Truth: There is a multitude of moisturizers available with different types of ingredients, purposes, and outcomes. Humectants, such as glycerin and lactic acid, attract water and help skin retain moisture. Emollients, such as fatty acids and ceramides, soften and soothe. Occlusives such as petrolatum, dimethicone or lanolin, leave a film on the surface of the skin and seal in moisture. Most products contain a combination of humectants, emollients and occlusives. Moisturizer is chosen based on the skin type—oily or acne-prone skin, sensitive skin, or dry skin; and climate—warm, dry or cold. Occlusives tend to be heavy while lotions are light, and creams are a little more substantial. For dry or extra-dry skin, it is better to use a cream which tends to protect skin better than lotion. Skin tends to be drier in colder months, so a cream should be used in winter, and a lotion in warmer weather.[2]

Box 1: Myths and misconceptions about moisturizers

- Oily skin does not need moisturizing
- All moisturizers are essentially the same
- Same moisturizer can be used for different body parts
- Creams are more efficacious moisturizers than lotions
- If moisturizer contains sunscreen, you do not need any other protection
- All cases of facial dryness need to be moisturized
- A topical medicine serves as both an active drug and a moisturizer
- Only ceramides can repair a disrupted skin barrier
- The ratio of ceramides within a moisturizer is important
- Prescription-barrier creams have superior efficacy to over-the-counter therapeutic moisturizers.
- "Natural" products are better
- Older, more common ingredients are not efficacious
- The myth of lanolin allergy
- Expensive moisturizers containing collagen can replace the collagen lost during the aging process
- Creams containing hyaluronic acid prolong the effect of hyaluronic acid fillers and have some antiwrinkle effect
- Moisturizers are safe and do not have any side effects.

Myth: Same moisturizer can be used for different body parts.
Truth: Many moisturizers can be used on most of the body; however the facial skin has special needs. It is rich in sebaceous glands, is exposed to sun and more prone to acne. Hence, it needs an oil-free moisturizer. For extremities which are dry and cracked, substantial creams are required.

Myth: Creams are more efficacious moisturizers than lotions.
Truth: Creams are thicker emulsion systems than lotions; however, they do not necessarily contain higher concentration of the active ingredient(s) or offer better protection against transepidermal water loss.

The efficacy of the moisturizer is determined by the efficacy of the humectants, occlusive and other agents that repair skin barrier. Further, lighter-weight lotions are being designed which have superior efficacy, are more pleasing to use and promote patient compliance.

Myth: If moisturizer contains sunscreen, you do not need any other protection.
Truth: There is a plethora of skincare and cosmetic products that have added sunscreen.

As long as the sunscreen has a sun protection factor (SPF) of 30 or higher and is a broad-spectrum sunscreen, which protects against both ultraviolet A (UVA) and ultraviolet B (UVB) rays, a separate sunscreen need not be applied. It may be wiser to have a separate moisturizer and sunscreen.

Myth: All cases of facial dryness need to be moisturized.
Truth: All patients with dryness on their face may not be having a true dry skin with low levels of sebum production, but a skin which appears dry because of lack of hydration. This distinction becomes very important in selecting the right type of moisturizers. True dry skin needs to be kept moisturized at all times as the sebaceous glands are not producing enough oil. Exfoliation is also important

to keep the dead cell buildup to a minimum. On the other hand, dehydration means there is hyperkeratosis, which renders the skin unable to retain water efficiently. To reduce or eliminate dehydration, regular and thorough exfoliation is required and overmoisturization will in fact worsen the condition by interfering with exfoliation.

Myth: A topical medicine serves as both an active drug and a moisturizer.
Truth: Medicinal creams and lotions contain penetration enhancers that open up the stratum corneum to allow penetration of the medicine to achieve the desired clinical effect. Thus, they disrupt the skin barrier, causing more water loss.[3] In order to support and improve the barrier condition, moisturizers need to be used as adjunctive therapy to optimize therapeutic outcomes.

Myth: Only ceramides can repair a disrupted skin barrier.
Truth: Adding ceramides to a topical formulation is not the only way to repair a disrupted barrier, since there are other factors too which help to repair the barrier function. Ingredients such as lactic acid and urea have been shown to stimulate endogenous ceramide production.[4,5] Acidic product formulations that preserve the acid mantle or hydrophobic ingredients like cholesterol and fatty acids which restore the barrier by protective effect also strengthen the skin's repair mechanisms to restore barrier health.

Myth: The ratio of ceramides within a moisturizer is important.
Truth: The ideal ratio of ceramide classes within healthy skin or in efficacious moisturizers is controversial.[1]

Myth: Prescription barrier creams have superior efficacy to over-the-counter therapeutic moisturizers.
Truth: Several studies have shown that over-the-counter quality therapeutic moisturizers have a comparable efficacy to medical device barrier creams.[6,7] Moreover, they are usually more cost effective.

Myth: "Natural" products are better.
Truth: There are no guidelines regarding what is a natural product. Natural extracts are not a single purified component but often are complex concentrates with trace amounts of unintended components. Therefore, their composition depends on the supplier and the manufacturing process.[8]

Myth: Older, more common ingredients are not efficacious.
Truth: New ingredients appear promising and more efficacious, purportedly overcoming the drawbacks of older ingredients. However, older agents have demonstrated efficacy and safety. Hence, before discarding time-tested formulations, the dermatologist should always demand clinical evidence of safety and efficacy of the new agents.

Myth: The myth of lanolin allergy.[9]
Truth: Lanolin has the reputation of being an important contact sensitizer and several products are labeled "lanolin free". In fact, pure lanolin is a weak sensitizer and lanolin-sensitive patients often are patch test negative to pure lanolin. This "lanolin paradox" was described by Wolff in 1996.[10] Lanolin is a natural product obtained from sheep fleece that contains complex mixture of esters and polyesters of high molecular weight alcohols and fatty acids, and

is an occlusive agent.[10] Ultra-pure medical grade lanolin products have been developed which are have minimal allergic potential.[2]

Myth: Expensive moisturizers containing collagen can replace the collagen lost during the aging process.
Truth: Only substances with a molecular weight of 5,000 Daltons or less can penetrate the stratum corneum whereas most of the collagen "extracts" have a molecular weight of 15,000–50,000 Daltons. At the most, they leave a film on the skin that fills in surface irregularities. Once the product dries, the protein films shrink slightly causing a subtle stretching out of fine skin wrinkles. Addition of humectants to these creams further plumps out the tiny wrinkles, thus giving a firming effect, albeit temporary.[2]

Myth: Creams containing hyaluronic acid (HA) prolong the effect of HA fillers and have some antiwrinkle effect.
Truth: Contrary to many marketing claims, HA cannot penetrate the epidermis and enter the dermis when applied topically. It only functions as a humectant on the skin's surface.[2]

Myth: Moisturizers are safe and do not have any side effects.
Truth: Generally, moisturizers are safe with few reports of side effects. However, allergic contact dermatitis can result from the use of preservatives, perfumes, solubilizers, sunscreens, and other skin care product constituents like vitamin E, propylene glycol and Kathon CG.[2]

Moisturizers are an important part of the dermatologist's armamentarium. Hence, it is essential to be aware of the different types of moisturizers as well as their properties, functions and ingredients. This knowledge will aid in their correct usage and help in separating myth from reality.

REFERENCES

1. Draelos ZD. Modern moisturizer myths, misconceptions, and truths. Cutis. 2013;91(6):308-14.
2. Baumann L. Moisturizing agents. In: Baumann L, Saghari S, Weisberg E (Eds). Cosmetic Dermatology: Principles and Practice, 2nd edition. New York: McGraw Hill; 2011. pp. 273-8.
3. Benson HA. Transdermal drug delivery: penetration enhancement techniques. Curr Drug Deliv. 2005;2(1):23-33.
4. Matts PJ, Rawlings AV. The dry skin cycle. In: Draelos ZD, Thaman LA (Eds). Cosmetic Formulation of Skin Care Products. New York, NY: Taylor & Francis Group; 2006. pp. 79-107.
5. Grether-Beck S, Felsner I, Brenden H, et al. Urea uptake enhances barrier function and antimicrobial defense in humans by regulating epidermal gene expression. J Invest Dermatol. 2012;132(6):1561-72.
6. Sarnoff DS. A comparison of wound healing between a skin protectant ointment and a medical device topical emulsion after laser resurfacing of the perioral area. J Am Acad Dermatol. 2011;64(3):S36-S43.
7. Miller DW, Koch SB, Yentzer BA, et al. An over-the-counter moisturizer is as clinically effective as, and more cost-effective than, prescription barrier creams in the treatment of children with mild-to-moderate atopic dermatitis: a randomized, controlled trial. J Drugs Dermatol. 2011;10:531-7.
8. Mukta S, Adam F. Cosmeceuticals in day-to-day clinical practice. J Drugs Dermatol. 2010;9(suppl 5):s62-6.
9. Kligman AM. The myth of lanolin allergy. Contact Dermatitis. 1998;39(3):103-7.
10. Matiz C, Jacob SE. The lanolin paradox revisited. J Am Acad Dermatol. 2011;64(1):197.

CHAPTER 3

Skin Barrier, Stratum Corneum Maturation, and Moisturization

Aayushi Mehta, Rashmi Sarkar

"The stratum corneum is a magnificent example of the successful adaptation of a tissue. Its efficient function is a prerequisite for life itself."

–Ronald Marks, Gerd Plewig

SKIN BARRIER

The epidermis or integument is the structure which protects us from various mechanical, physical, and infectious stimuli in the environment. In addition, it serves the very important function of preventing water loss and maintaining adequate skin hydration. The epidermis prevents prevents external agents from entering the body, and prevents water and polar compounds from evaporating from the surface. Thus, it is often called the "skin barrier", in referral to its primary and most essential function in our bodies.

DISCOVERY IN HISTORY

We now know that the human skin is a highly evolved organ with a multiplicity of functions. In the 1950s, the stratum corneum (SC), or the horny layer, was thought to be an amorphous, acellular, disorganized mass of keratins, produced by the cells of the basal layer of the epidermis. Albert Kligman in 1964 demonstrated that the SC was a cellular structure made of cells which he labeled as "corneocytes". Thus, it was proven that the histopathological image of the SC, that histopathologists had been seeing as the "basket-weave" pattern, was in fact an artifact due to formalin fixation.[1]

The barrier function of the skin started receiving much attention. Initially, the skin barrier was thought to reside at the stratum corneum-stratum granulosum interface.[2] However, it was soon proven that the entire SC was the site of "the barrier".[3]

The "brick and mortar" model of the epidermis was first described by Peter Elias and his coworkers.[4] The corneocytes containing hydrophilic keratin correlated to the bricks and the intercellular hydrophobic lamellar lipid correlated to the mortar. Thus, this two compartment model was composed of lipid-depleted cells surrounded by a lipid-enriched intercellular domain, and this was thought to be the actual site of the physical barrier in our skin (Figure 1).

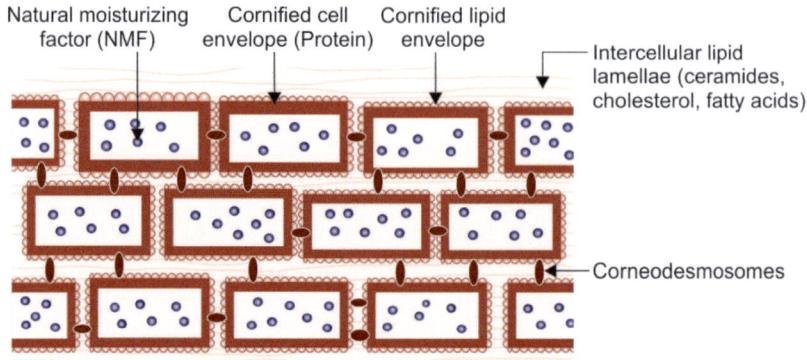

Figure 1: A schematic representation of the brick and mortar model of the stratum corneum.

It is now apparent that the intercellular spaces of the SC enclose lipid membrane bilayers which participate in the barrier function.[3]

Later, studies have proved even this model to be an oversimplification of the very complex organization of the SC.

The normal lipid composition in the skin barrier is 40% ceramides, 25% fatty acids, almost 20% cholesterol and 2–3% of components like cholesterol sulfate, phospholipids and triglycerides. Alteration in any of these components creates a defective water barrier function.

ROLE OF LAMELLAR BODIES AND MATURATION OF STRATUM CORNEUM

Lamellar bodies are unique, ovoid, membrane-covered secretory organelles produced by keratinocytes. They are also called as Odland bodies (after George Odland)/cementosomes/keratinosomes/membrane-coating granules.[5,6] They play an integral role in the formation of the epidermal permeability barrier.

Severe reduction or absence of lamellar bodies is seen in Harlequin ichthyosis,[6] which results in total disruption of normal skin barrier and high mortality. Thus, these small organelles are vital for maintenance of life.

The uppermost layer of the stratum granulosum (SG) synthesizes and secretes lamellar bodies. A variety of important functions have been described for these bodies including cohesion of keratinocytes, regulation of keratinocyte desquamation, cornification, skin barrier formation, hydration and antimicrobial actions.[3]

The lamellar bodies are first secreted at the level of the SG, initially containing precursors and probarrier polar lipids (glucosylceramides, cholesterol sulfate, glycerophospholipids, sphingomyelin). They also contain various requisite lipid processing enzymes and other additional proteins. At the SG-SC junction, the lamellar body migrates to the apex of the granular cell and secretes its disk like contents into the intercellular space.[7] At this stage, these probarrier lipids undergo maturation/conversion into non-polar, neutral lipids by enzyme action (hydrolysis). These are now remodeled as parallel broad laminae in the lower SC, participating in the permeability barrier.[5]

Exocytosis of lamellar bodies is the mechanism by which cells of epidermis deliver lipids and lipid-processing enzymes to the extracellular spaces of the SC. The intercellular lamellae are now composed of ceramides, free fatty acids, and cholesterol, which are the normal components of the intact skin barrier.[8]

The SC contains a lipid layer that is covalently attached to proteins on the external surface of the corneocytes (the corneocyte protein envelope). This lipid layer forms the "corneocyte lipid envelope". The intercellular lipid lamellae get attached to this envelope and these together form the permeability barrier.[9]

Soaps and surfactants make the skin barrier weaker as they leach ceramides from the skin surface. Various other environmental agents such as excessive use of hot or cold water, chemical exposure, pollution, all contribute to disruption of the intact skin barrier. In conditions where this barrier is disturbed, there will be increased secretion of lamellar bodies along with increased synthesis as well. Deficiency of extracellular calcium has also been known to promote secretion of lamellar bodies.

STRATUM CORNEUM HYDRATION

While the most important function of the SC is to maintain an impermeable barrier and prevent water loss from the body to the environment, it does allow a small amount of water loss to its outermost layers in order to maintain hydration. Adequate hydration of corneocytes is essential to maintain flexibility and functionality.

NATURAL MOISTURIZING FACTOR

Corneocytes contain certain hygroscopic compounds/osmolyte proteins called natural moisturizing factors (NMFs). These play a central role in mediating and maintaining epidermal tissue hydration and flexibility.

As water is constantly lost from skin surface by diffusion and evaporation, various mechanisms are at play in the skin to maintain homeostasis and adequate hydration in all the layers including the outermost, that is, the SC.

Three different types of water have been described in the SC: (1) Primary bound water—water tightly bound to SC proteins (seen at <10% hydration); (2) secondary bound water—water less tightly bound, that is, bound to corneocyte osmolytes and to the primary bound water (at 10–40% hydration) and (3) bulk liquid water (at 50% hydration).[10]

Occlusion greatly increases the local hydration in SC, leading to formation of frank extracellular pools of water.[11] There is production of spaces termed as "lacunae" within the intercellular mortar lipids.[3] A transient interconnection between these lacunae may allow increased passage of both hydrophilic and hydrophobic compounds, thus elucidating the mechanism for increased penetration of medications such as topical steroids after hydration.

Studies have shown that there are water gradients at different levels in the skin, due to presence of water in different concentrations at different levels. This variation in water content in the different layers is seen as follows: 15% at the skin surface, 40% at the innermost layer of the SC, and 80% within the granular

Table 1: Contents of natural moisturizing factor with their concentrations[11]

Natural moisturizing factor components	Concentration (%)
Amino acids	40
Pyrrolidone carboxylic acid	12
Lactate	12
Urea	7
Electrolytes (sodium, chloride, potassium)	15
Calcium, magnesium, phosphate	3.5
Sugars	8.5
Others	2

layer. Thus, there seems to be a discontinuity or barrier to water loss at the SC-granular interface.[11]

Stratum corneum NMF consists of amino acids and their derivatives, mainly being pyrrolidone carboxylic acid (PCA), lactic acid, urea, citrate, chloride, etc. Table 1 gives the contents of NMF with their concentrations.[11]

Natural moisturizing factor has both intra- and extracellular components and it is intensely hygroscopic in nature. Thus, it helps to ensure that even the outermost layers of the SC remain hydrated, despite environmental humidity and temperature variations.

Amino acids and their derivatives within the SC represent more than 50% of NMF. These are derived from their precursors—profilaggrin and filaggrin. Profilaggrin is first expressed in the granular layer cells. During the formation of corneocytes from granular cells, profilaggrin is converted to filaggrin. Filaggrin itself undergoes proteolysis in corneocytes to form NMF. The concentration of water in the SC itself in turn regulates the rate of formation of this NMF, thus completing the cycle.

TRANSEPIDERMAL WATER LOSS

Transepidermal water loss (TEWL) has been defined as the constitutive steady state water loss from the skin surface. This has been considered to occur due to passive diffusion, excluding water loss due to sweating. The SC forms the most important rate limiting step to this process.[12]

Evidence suggests that when there is injury or damage to the epidermal barrier, there is increased TEWL. This increased TEWL in turn promotes and upregulates the synthesis of barrier lipids, leading to restoration of the disrupted barrier.[13] Transepidermal water loss measurements are often used to study the integrity of the skin barrier and measurement of disease activity in conditions such as atopic dermatitis, ichthyosis and psoriasis.

Thus, application of external creams containing substances such as ceramides, help to restore the physical barrier of the skin, reduce the water loss, improve skin hydration, and eventually disrupt the cycle causing dry, itchy skin in various disease states.

Dry skin is noted clinically when there is an increased TEWL and inadequate hydration of SC. Minimum 10% of water is needed in the SC for the skin to be supple. Hydration up to 25–35% is preferred. However, when hydration falls below 10%, skin becomes very dry producing symptoms such as scaling and pruritus.

There is much regional difference in the rates of TEWL in the skin measured over different anatomic sites, probably because, in addition to maintaining skin homeostasis, TEWL also has other functions such as temperature regulation.

Thus, SC hydration not only has a role in maintaining skin flexibility, but it also participates in a variety of other functions, such as generation of NMF, lipid processing and barrier formation, corneodesmolysis and desquamation, etc.

CONCLUSION

It is now clear that the human epidermis and SC are complex organ systems with varied functions, and have multiple mechanisms for self-preservation and recovery following environmental damage. All these mechanism come together and result in the environmental adaptability of humans, survival in harsh climates and maintenance of the disease-free state of the epidermis.

REFERENCES

1. Kligman AM. A brief history of how the dead stratum corneum became alive. In: Elias PM, Feingold KR (Eds). Skin Barrier. New York: Taylor & Francis Group; 2006. pp. 15-24.
2. Elias PM. Epidermal lipids, membranes, and keratinization. Int J Dermatol. 1981;20(1):1-19.
3. Menon GK, Kligman AM. Barrier functions of human skin: a holistic view. Skin Pharmacol Physiol. 2009;22(4):178-89.
4. Elias PM, Feingold KR. Permeability barrier homeostasis. In: Elias PM, Feingold KR (Eds). Skin Barrier. New York: Taylor & Francis; 2006. pp. 337-62.
5. Elias PM, Grayson S, Lampe MA, et al. The intercorneocyte space. In: Marks R, Plewig G (Eds). Stratum Corneum. New York: Springer-Verlag Berlin Heidelberg; 1983. pp. 53-67.
6. Elias PM, Feingold KR, Fartasch M. The epidermal lamellar body as a multifunctional secretory organelle. In: Elias PM, Feingold KR (Eds). Skin Barrier. New York: Taylor & Francis Group; 2006. pp. 261-72.
7. Judge MR, McLean WH, Munro CS. Disorders of keratinization. In: Burns T, Breathnach S, Cox N, Griffiths C (Eds). Rook's Textbook of Dermatology, 8th edition (Volume 1). UK: Blackwell Science Ltd; 2010. pp. 19.1-19.122.
8. Wertz PW. Biochemistry of human stratum corneum lipids. In: Elias PM, Feingold KR (Eds). Skin Barrier. New York: Taylor & Francis Group; 2006. pp. 33-42.
9. Koch PJ, Roop DR, Zhou Z. Cornified envelope and corneocyte-lipid envelope. In: Elias PM, Feingold KR (Eds). Skin Barrier. New York: Taylor & Francis Group; 2006. pp. 97-110.
10. Idson B. Water & the skin. J Soc Cosmet Chem. 1973;24:197-212.
11. Rawlings AV. Sources and role of stratum corneum hydration. In: Elias PM, Feingold KR (Eds). Skin Barrier. New York: Taylor & Francis Group; 2006. pp. 399-426.
12. van der Valk PG, Kucharekova M, Tupker RA. Transepidermal water loss and its relation to barrier function and skin irritation. In: Fluhr J, Elsner P, Berardesca E, Maibach HI (Eds). Bioengineering of the Skin: Water and the Stratum Corneum, 2nd edition. USA: CRC Press; 2005. pp. 97-104.
13. Grubauer G, Elias PM, Feingold KR. Transepidermal water loss: the signal for recovery of barrier structure and function. J Lipid Res. 1989;30(3):323-33.

CHAPTER 4

Indications of Moisturizers in Skin

Pooja Arora

INTRODUCTION

Moisturizers are required for the daily maintenance of normal skin and are the mainstay of treatment for dry skin. They are also used as adjunctive therapy for many skin diseases characterized by xerosis and impaired skin barrier. In this chapter we will discuss the indications of moisturizers on skin (Table 1).

DRY SKIN (XEROSIS CUTIS)

Dry skin is characterized by a rough or scaly appearance of skin with an irregular feel on touch. Cracking and reddening may be associated with dry skin. There is increase in skin markings and erythematous lines can develop with time. The sites most affected are the lower legs, dorsal aspect of forearms and hands. Dry skin can lead to pruritus and eczema. People with dry skin have a genetic predisposition to it. Systemic diseases like hypothyroidism, uremia, diabetes as well as certain medications like isotretinoin can lead to dry skin. Treatment of xerosis is aimed at restoration of the epidermal barrier with liberal use of moisturizers. Application of emollients immediately after bath improves the hydration of the stratum corneum (SC). Moisturizers make the skin smooth as they fill the gaps between the desquamated corneocytes. They also reduce the friction on the skin. Studies have shown that moisturizers reduce the soap-induced xerosis.[1]

Table 1: Indications of moisturizers on skin

Indications	
Dry skin (xerosis)	Genetic, associated with systemic diseases (hypothyroidism, uremia, diabetes, chronic illness), medications (isotretinoin, lithium)
Eczema	Asteatotic eczema, atopic dermatitis, hand eczema
Disorders of keratinization	Ichthyosis, keratoderma, psoriasis
Acne	Acne treated with retinoids, rosacea
Aging	Chronic pruritus in elderly, atrophic vaginitis, photoaged skin
Miscellaneous	Scars and striae

Alpha or beta hydroxy acids are special moisturizing agents that promote corneocyte desquamation, and hence decrease roughness. These are also helpful in the treatment of photoaged skin.

ECZEMA

Moisturizers are the mainstay of treatment of asteatotic eczema. They are also used for the treatment and prevention of hand eczema. Patients with hand eczema should apply emollients (humectants and lipids) liberally to hands after work. It should be noted that urea in moisturizers can increase skin permeability to irritants and should be avoided.[2] White petrolatum is a purified derivative of mineral oil and consists of long chained aliphatic hydrocarbons. Studies have shown that white petrolatum protects the skin from water-soluble skin irritants. It also hastens barrier recovery. Hence, it serves both as an effective moisturizer as well as a barrier cream and is the topical emollient of choice in hand eczema.

Moisturizers can also decrease the inflammation in damaged and irritated skin. Loden and colleagues studied the effects of topically applied lipids on surfactant irritated skin and found that moisturizers containing canola oil can reduce irritation induced by sodium lauryl sulfate (SLS) as they supply the damaged barrier with adequate lipids.[3]

ATOPIC DERMATITIS

Moisturizers provide numerous benefits in patients with atopic dermatitis (AD). They increase the hydration of the SC by occluding the skin surface which reduces the water loss. The addition of humectants in moisturizers amplifies their hydrating power by attracting and holding water. Humectants widely used are glycerin, lactic acid, urea and pyrrolidone carboxylic acid (PCA). Studies have shown that humectants help to maintain the bilayer lipids of skin in a liquid crystalline state at low humidity.

Moisturizers also improve the abnormal barrier function of skin in patients with atopic eczema. They relieve the pruritus, hence reducing scratching. They increase the SC elasticity by improving the skin hydration. Hence, the risk of cracking and barrier disruption is reduced. Lipids such as petrolatum are absorbed into the outer layer of delipidized SC.

"Physiologic" lipids can even modify endogenous epidermal lipids and the rate of barrier recovery. Moisturizers can also have anti-inflammatory effects. The essential fatty acids (EFAs), which are an important component of the epidermal phospholipids, are incorporated in ceramics and play role in barrier function. EFA influences eicosanoid production, membrane fluidity and cell signaling. Few ingredients of moisturizers have antimicrobial properties. One such component is propylene glycol that has antifungal properties and inhibits growth of *Trichophyton*, *Malassezia* and *Candida*.[4]

Use of moisturizers in patients with AD not only increases the hydration of the skin but also lessens symptoms and signs of AD. Randomized controlled trials (RCTs) have shown that use of moisturizers decreases the amount of anti-inflammatory agents (especially corticosteroids) required for control of diseases.[5] American Academy of Dermatology (AAD) guidelines recommend moisturizers as the main primary treatment for mild disease, and as a part of the treatment regimen for moderate and severe disease.[6] They are also an important part of the maintenance treatment and help to prevent flares of AD. The optimal amount or frequency of application of moisturizers has not been defined due to lack of studies. However, it is recommended that moisturizers be applied frequently (at least twice a day) and in liberal amount to reduce xerosis.

Adults should generally be using 500–600 g per week and children 250 mg per week. One set of guidelines recommends that the amount of emollient used should exceed steroid use by a ratio of 10:1. Moisturizers should be applied liberally all over the body, not just on localized areas of dry skin. They should be applied after bath or shower to help retain the hydration. Application of emollients and steroids should be separated by 30 minutes. This period should be 1 hour for tacrolimus. Patients should not insert hands or fingers into emollient pots in order to avoid microbial contamination of contents. There are hundreds of moisturizers available in market and it is difficult for the dermatologist to choose the right product. Important considerations should be the ingredient, tolerability and patient preference. The patient can be offered a number of choices and allowed to choose the one that suits them the most. Patients may require more than one emollient product depending on lifestyle, time of day, seasonal factors or disease severity. When choosing moisturizers for AD it is important to remember that they cannot cure flare of AD and should be appropriately combined with anti-inflammatory agents. Intermittent use of antiseptic bath oils can reduce the flares.

In the last few years, a newer class of topical agents has been designed for the treatment of AD. These are the prescription emollient devices (PEDs). They target the specific defects in skin barrier function seen in patients with AD. Their composition mimics the endogenous lipids and they may also contain palmitoylethanolamide, glycyrrhetinic acid and other lipids. There are very few studies regarding the use of PED, but there is evidence that they lessen the xerosis and inflammation in AD.

ICHTHYOSIS

Moisturizers form an important component of topical treatment of ichthyoses. Bathing followed by application of moisturizer improves the skin hydration. Patients with thick and dense scales may benefit with lukewarm baths and showers with short to moderate soak times.[7] Bath additives can be used to provide additional moisturization. Mineral oil can be used both as a topical moisturizer and as a bath oil. Patients should be cautious when using bath oils as they are slippery.

The choice of moisturizer depends on the patient's preference. White petrolatum jelly is one of the most widely used moisturizer and is readily available in the market. It should be used with caution around open flames as it is flammable. Newer moisturizers containing ceramides that are deficient in affected skin are available nowadays.

The potential disadvantage of the formulation should be kept in mind when prescribing moisturizers. Ointments may be superior to creams but are greasier and more occlusive. They also tend to be messier and give a shiny appearance to skin. They can stain the clothing and bedding. Patients using ointments during summer months may feel hotter as ointments are more occlusive. This can be avoided by refrigerating the ointment before using. During cold environments, ointments tend to become stiff and creams may be better tolerated. One disadvantage of creams is that they require preservatives to prevent bacterial overgrowth as they have relatively high water content. This can increase the risk of allergic contact dermatitis with the creams. Patients with ichthyosis need to be told about the requirement of a large amount of moisturizer and lifelong application.

Moisturizers containing humectants can be helpful in patients with ichthyosis. Alpha hydroxy acids, propylene glycol, urea, glycerin, hyaluronic acid are the ones readily available. Glycerin is a readily available humectant that can be applied directly onto the skin as well as hair-bearing areas. It is more cosmetically appealing as it is less greasy. Urea is also a component of moisturizers. It is also available as a 20% or 40% cream. The latter is especially helpful in areas with thick and dense scales. Caution should be exercised when using urea in infants and young children with ichthyosis as urea can get absorbed leading to elevated plasma blood urea nitrogen levels.[8]

PSORIASIS

Use of moisturizers offer several benefits in patients with psoriasis. Regular use of moisturizers improves comfort and reduces scaling, fissuring and itching. Emollients enhance the penetration of CS through the skin, and hence may increase the efficacy of the latter. However, the steroid-sparing effects of emollients is yet to be proven as RCTs have shown inconsistent results.[9,10]

It has been proposed that emollient monotherapy in psoriasis may improve skin hydration, barrier function as well as proliferation and differentiation markers. However, clinical trials have shown only limited evidence in this regard and need evaluation through larger trials.

Few studies have shown that some moisturizers (e.g., oil-in-water emollient) enhance the penetration of ultraviolet A (UVA) or ultraviolet B (UVB) when used before irradiation, and thus can increase the efficacy of phototherapy.[11] On the contrary, few *in vitro* studies and trials in healthy volunteers have shown a blocking effect of few emollients (e.g., white petrolatum).[12] However, practice shows that white soft petrolatum is a good moisturizer in psoriasis and can be used after topical coal tar and in conjunction with dithranol or topical steroids. It will have a good steroid-sparing effect.

Urea-containing preparations form an important component of adjuvant therapy of psoriasis. Urea offers multiple benefits. It reduces the epidermal hyperproliferation and induces cell differentiation. *In vitro* and *in vivo* studies have found that application of urea causes reduction of DNA synthesis in cells of the basal layers, and thinning of the epidermis and prolongs the generation time of postmitotic cells. Urea disperses and denatures keratin by breaking the hydrogen bonds and interfering with its quaternary structure. Urea also enhances the efficacy of other topical therapies when used concomitantly. Thus, urea is a preferred moisturizer in patients with psoriasis.

To summarize, moisturizers can be effective in removing scales before active treatments are used. They also have anti-inflammatory and antikeratotic effects.

ACNE

Dimethicone and glycerin are common ingredients of moisturizers used in patients of acne. Dimethicone is usually used in "oil free" moisturizers. The latter do not contain mineral or vegetable oil. Dimethicone has both occlusive and emollient properties and reduces transepidermal water loss (TEWL). It does not have a greasy feel and is noncomedogenic and hypoallergenic. Mineral oil is comedogenic and is usually not a component of moisturizers used for acne. However, cosmetic grade mineral oil may be used as it is noncomedogenic.

Dimethicone is generally combined with glycerin in acne moisturizers. Glycerin is a humectant but when used alone can increase TEWL. Therefore, it is usually combined with an occlusive agent. Ingredients like aloe vera and allantoin are added in the moisturizers for their anti-inflammatory properties. Aloe vera inhibits cyclooxygenase in the arachidonic pathway causing anti-inflammatory properties. However, it should be present at a concentration of at least 10% in order to have a moisturizing effect.[13]

Trials have shown that the adjunctive use of a moisturizer improves local tolerance of topical retinoids. Study performed by Hayashi, et al. has shown that the combined use of moisturizers with adapalene form the beginning of treatment and is useful in reducing the rate of discontinuation of treatment due to the adverse reactions to the drug.[14] Topical retinoids have been associated with adverse effects like skin discomfort, dry skin and exfoliation. Continued use of the drug reduces the frequency of these adverse reactions. However, patients might discontinue treatment once adverse effects occur.

CHRONIC PRURITUS IN ELDERLY

Moisturizers are the mainstay of treatment of pruritus in the elderly, especially in patients associated with xerosis. They improve the skin barrier function by preventing TEWL and by preventing the entry of irritants into the skin. This causes relief in pruritus. Moisturizers with low pH should be used to maintain the normal acidic pH of the skin surface. Studies have shown that serine proteases, via protease-activating receptor (PAR)-2 located on C-fiber terminals, play an important role in mediating pruritus. Low pH topical treatments reduce the activity of serine proteases (e.g., mast cell tryptase) that activate PAR-2 on skin nerve fibers.

ATROPHIC VAGINITIS

Physiologic and structural changes occur within the vulvovaginal mucosa with menopause due to the loss of estrogen. This leads to atrophic vaginitis causing vulvovaginal dryness, vulvar itching or pain, dyspareunia and abnormal vaginal discharge. Vaginal moisturizers can provide symptomatic relief for vaginal dryness in this condition. They can be used on a chronic, maintenance basis to replace normal vaginal secretions. The most widely used ingredient in such vaginal moisturizers is polycarbophil, which is a bioadhesive polymer that adheres to the vaginal walls after application and releases water and electrolytes into the epithelium, thereby making the surface moist. Polycarbophil also causes vasodilation by inducing migration of water and electrolytes into the dermal vasculature. This in turn leads to improved tissue hydration. It has a pH of 2.8, hence shifts the pH of the vagina to more acidic premenopausal state. Studies have shown that such vaginal moisturizers can reduce symptoms of atrophic vaginitis and are a good alternative in females with contraindication to estrogen.

SCARS AND STRIAE

Scars and striae have a malfunctional SC that has increased TEWL and reduced capacitance. Occlusion therapy is known to improve the signs and symptoms of scarring. However, apart from the pressure-related effects, direct effects of hydration on keratinocytes and fibroblasts contribute to the reduction in hypertrophic scarring. Occlusion can also cause changes in epidermal cytokines and growth factor production causing changes in fibrotic factors. Several studies have shown that moisturizers reduce the clinical signs and symptoms of scars and striae.

THERAPEUTIC MOISTURIZERS

Specific ingredients can be added to moisturizers to enhance the therapeutic potential. Such "therapeutic moisturizers" are now readily available in the market.[15] Examples of such ingredients include alpha hydroxy acids, beta hydroxy acids and vitamins. Alpha hydroxy acids (glycolic and lactic acid) provide antiaging effect whereas beta hydroxy acids (salicylic acid) are components of exfoliant moisturizers. Topical vitamin C and vitamin E provide antioxidant effects whereas panthenol is a skin conditioning agent added to moisturizers for additional benefits.

REFERENCES

1. Olivarius FD, Hansen AB, Karlsmark T, et al. Water protective effect of barrier creams and moisturizing creams: a new in vivo test method. Contact Dermatitis. 1996;35(4):219-25.
2. Wohlrab W. The influence of urea on the penetration kinetics of topically applied corticosteroids. Acta Derm Venereol (Stockh). 1984;64(3):233-8.
3. Loden M, Andersson AC. Effects of topically applied lipids on surfactant-irritated skin. Brit J Dermatol. 1996;134(2):215-20.
4. Faergemann J, Fredriksson T. Antimycotic activity of propane-1, 2-diol (propylene glycol). Sabouraudia. 1980;18(3):163-9.
5. Grimalt R, Mengeaud V, Cambazard F, et al. The steroid-sparing effect of an emollient therapy in infants with atopic dermatitis: a randomized controlled study. Dermatology. 2007;214(1):61-7.
6. Eichenfield LF, Tom WL, Berger TG, et al. Guidelines of care for the management of atopic dermatitis: section 2. Management and treatment of atopic dermatitis with topical therapies. J Am Acad Dermatol. 2014;71(1):116-32.
7. Fleckman P, Newell BD, van Steensel MA, et al. Topical treatment of ichthyoses. Dermatol Ther. 2013;26(1):16-25.
8. Garty BZ. High plasma urea concentration in babies with lamellar ichthyosis. Arch Dis Child. 1986;61(12):1245-6.
9. Tanghetti EA, Tazarotene Stable Plaque Psoriasis Trial Study Group. An observation study evaluating the treatment of plaque psoriasis with tazarotene gels, alone and with an emollient and/or corticosteroid. Cutis. 2000;66(6 suppl):4-11.

10. Watsky KL, Freije L, Leneveu MC, et al. Water-in-oil emollients as steroid-sparing adjunctive therapy in the treatment of psoriasis. Cutis. 1992;50(5):383-6.
11. Boyvat A, Erdi H, Birol A, et al. Interaction of commonly used emollients with photochemotherapy. Photodermatol Photoimmunol Photomed. 2000;16(4):156-60.
12. Kristensen B, Kristensen O. Topical salicylic acid interferes with UVB therapy for psoriasis. Acta Derm Venereol. 1991;71(1):37-40.
13. Chularojanamontri L, Tuchinda P, Kulthanan K, et al. Moisturizers for acne: What are their constituents? J Clin Aesthet Dermatol. 2014;7(5):36-44.
14. Hayashi N, Kawashima M. Study of the usefulness of moisturizers on adherence of acne patients treated with adapalene. J Dermatol. 2014;41(7):592-7.
15. Draelos ZD. Therapeutic moisturizers. Derm Clin. 2000;18(4):597-607.

CHAPTER 5

Moisturizers in Atopic Dermatitis

Sumit Sethi

INTRODUCTION

Atopic dermatitis (AD) (with a synonym of atopic eczema or "eczema") is a common chronic inflammatory skin disease with increasing prevalence. The pathophysiology is multifactorial, probably involves an interaction of both environmental and genetic factors which cause abnormalities in the epidermal barrier and the immune system. Both phenotypes, the barrier-initiated mechanism (outside-inside hypothesis) and the primary immunological abnormality mechanism (inside-outside hypothesis) have similar skin lesions and distribution patterns. AD is characterized by exacerbations and remissions and need a multifaceted treatment strategy.[1,2]

ABNORMAL EPIDERMAL BARRIER IN THE PATHOGENESIS OF ATOPIC DERMATITIS

There is now scientific evidence of genetically driven skin barrier anomalies in atopic patients. Abnormal proteins (filaggrin), lack of stratum corneum intercellular lipids and an inadequate ratio between compounds (cholesterol, essential fatty acids, ceramides), together with a protease-antiprotease imbalance, are responsible for the complex AD pathophysiology. The barrier anomalies facilitate sustained antigen penetration and enhanced transepidermal water loss, leading to the release of preformed proinflammatory cytokines and to a cascade of events ending up in inflammation (Th2-dominant response). Successful treatment requires a holistic approach that consists of avoidance of triggering factors, optimal skin care, pharmacotherapy during acute exacerbations, and education of patients/caregivers.[3,4]

ROLE OF MOISTURIZERS IN ATOPIC DERMATITIS

The skin barrier dysfunction plays a prominent role in the development and perpetuation of AD, the "outside-to-inside" view of AD pathogenesis. With dry skin (xerosis) being one of the cardinal features of AD, and part of its definition, moisturizers form the basic treatment for disturbed skin barrier (i.e., the preferred skin care therapy) (Figure 1).[1] Moisturizers combat xerosis and transepidermal

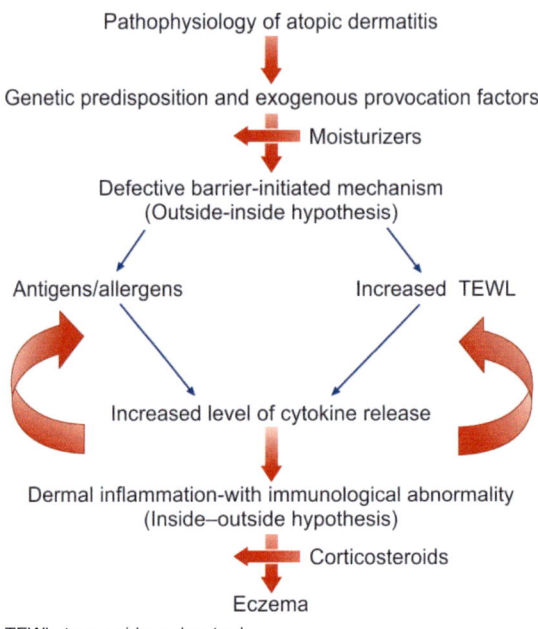

Figure 1: Defective skin barrier function increases skin susceptibility and triggers eczema.[7]

water loss, with traditional agents containing varying amounts of emollient, occlusive, and/or humectant ingredients. Although they often include water as well, this only delivers a transient effect, whereas the other components provide the main benefits. Emollients (e.g., glycol and glyceryl stearate, soy sterols) lubricate and soften the skin, occlusive agents (e.g., petrolatum, dimethicone, mineral oil) form a layer to retard evaporation of water, whereas humectants (e.g., glycerol, lactic acid, urea) attract and hold water. Moisturizers reduce scratching by helping to relieve the pruritus that characterizes AD. They play a pivotal role in improving and maintaining the skin barrier function and reducing skin susceptibility to irritants. Furthermore, increased skin hydration increase stratum corneum elasticity and reduce the risks of cracking and barrier disruption.[5] Regular use of emollients decreases the amount of prescription anti-inflammatory treatments (topical steroids and calcineurin inhibitors) required for disease in mild-to-moderate AD. They lessen symptoms and signs of AD, including pruritus, erythema, fissuring, and lichenification.[2,4]

What, When and How Much to Apply?

There is a paucity of data examining the optimal emollient and its amount or frequency of application for this condition. It is generally thought that liberal and frequent reapplication is necessary such that xerosis is minimal. Non-lesional AD skin looks normal to the naked eye, but harbors subclinical inflammation. Emollients should be recommended in adequate amounts and used liberally and frequently in atopic patients.[4] They should be applied after any topical pharmacologic therapies to allow active medications to reach the skin with full effect. Frequency of application of emollients/moisturizers may be more important than timing the application to coincide strictly with bathing (the traditional "soak and seal" approach). The traditional theory that emollients should be applied within 3 minutes after bath to retain hydration (3 minute rule), remains to be confirmed in larger, more controlled studies.[1]

Other important things to consider before prescribing an emollient are *tolerability and cost*. Although emollients are widely used and inexpensive in most cases, but there are ever increasing dangers of contact sensitization because of their complicated composition. Contact sensitization or irritation by components of the emollients/moisturizers may worsen the skin condition in AD and influence the course and the severity of eczema, especially by the use of complex composed moisturizers. Moreover, sensitized atopic subjects may respond to very low concentrations of contact allergens because of their impaired skin barrier function and hyper-reactivity to irritant stimuli enhancing contact reactions.[2] A possible solution suggested by Gelmetti is to apply two different products to either side of the body and then observe for any possible signs and symptoms for next 20 minutes. All possible acute intolerances or idiosyncrasies should present during this period and it will be easier to prescribe the right emollient for that patient and gain their adherence to treatment.[1]

Traditional moisturizers are formulated into a variety of delivery systems, including creams, ointments, oils, gels and lotions. With little evidence to recommend the use of one emollient/moisturizer over another, patient and caregiver preference should be considered with product selection based on the premise that "an emollient that is applied works better than one that remains on a shelf". Although most ointments have the advantage of not containing preservatives, which may cause stinging when applied to inflamed skin, they may be too greasy for some patients with AD. Very occlusive ointments may not be tolerated during the summer months or in humid climates because of interference with the function of eccrine sweat ducts and the induction of folliculitis; in these situations, a cream may be a more practical choice. Lotions have a higher water content that can evaporate and may be less ideal in those with significant xerosis. Also it is best to avoid preparations that contain topical sensitizers such as fragrance, neomycin, benzocaine, etc.[6]

It is important to remember that emollients and moisturizers cannot cure AD flares; in fact they can sometimes exacerbate AD when applied at the "wrong" moment (e.g., the sole use of emollients without sufficient topical anti-inflammatory therapy increases the risk of disseminated infections, which are already raised in patients with AD). After cessation of visible lesions, all anti-inflammatory therapy has to be tapered down and stopped completely in favor of an exclusive therapy with barrier-stabilizing emollients.[1]

Simple Oil-in-Water Emollients

Petrolatum-based emollients have been the workhorse for flare prevention in AD. The lipids found in petrolatum permeate the interstitial compartment of the stratum corneum and enhance the lipid barrier. It does not need preservatives or fragrances, improves barrier function and improve long-term control of the disease while reducing topical steroid use.[6]

BARRIER REPAIR THERAPEUTICS—CONTROVERSY?

In a state of physiologic balance, the approximate proportions of the lipid component are 50–60% ceramides, 15–25% cholesterol, and 10–20% free fatty acids (3:1:1). In AD, there is a decrease in all three key lipids, especially ceramides, which are found in both affected and non-affected skin.[4] A new concept in skin barrier care is the incorporation of balanced proportions of stratum corneum-specific lipids [natural moisturizing factors (NMFs), ceramides, and pseudoceramide products] into therapeutic moisturizers.[4] These, "barrier repair therapeutics" target specific defects in skin barrier function and have entered the market as prescription emollient devices (PEDs), i.e., "510(k)-cleared" devices, where the focus is on safety as opposed to efficacy. They are approved as 510(k) medical devices based on the assertion that they serve a structural role in skin barrier function and do not exert their effects by any chemical actions. This approval process requires less rigorous clinical efficacy data than that needed for Food and Drug Administration approval of drugs. They include preparations having distinct ratios of lipids that mimic endogenous compositions and creams containing palmitoylethanolamide, glycyrrhetinic acid, or other hydrolipids. These products contain ingredients that attempt to replace or correct deficiencies of epidermal lipids, improve skin hydration, reduce skin barrier dysfunction, and relieve the pruritus, burning and pain associated with AD. They are generally recommended for 2 or 3 times daily use depending on the specific agent. While there is some evidence that PEDs also lessen symptoms and signs of AD, including xerosis and inflammation, they have only been tested in a small number of controlled studies. In addition, these agents are more costly, although they are considered safe adjunctive treatments. There are now several moisturizers containing ceramides and/or filaggrin breakdown products that are available over-the-counter (OTC), though the compositions are not necessarily equivalent to those of the PEDs. Four products have been approved as 510(k) medical device creams by US FDA and are available over the past several years for the treatment of AD. These include EpiCeram® (Dr Reddy Laboratories), Atopiclair® (Menarini), Mimyx® containing lamellar matrix of pharmaceutical emollient palmitoylethanolamine (Steifel Laboratories–PEA now present in Physiogel) and Eletone® emulsion (Mission Pharmacal Company) (Table 1).[4,6]

Although this new class of moisturizers has shown excellent performance, efficacy, and safety, there is no scientific evidence to support their superiority over a well-crafted traditional, petrolatum-based OTC emollient. Head-to-head trials between specific moisturizing products are few in number, and those performed to date have not demonstrated one to be superior to others, including the PEDs. In addition, there is currently no definition for "barrier-repair products", which raises the question of whether presently available products could justify such a category.[4]

Current research on efficacy of their use appears conflicting and inconsistent. Some studies showed only mild improvement of severity or skin hydration, while others demonstrated moderate corticosteroid sparing effects. Many trials had very small sample sizes and did not evaluate all relevant clinical and biophysical parameters. Well designed, large-scale, randomized, placebo-controlled trials to document the therapeutic effects on disease severity, dermatologic biophysical

Table 1: Moisturizers for atopic dermatitis in India

Product	Other ingredients	Special/key ingredients
Physiogel cream	Ceramide, triglycerides, glycerin, squalane, hydrogenated lecithin	–
Physiogel lotion	Ceramide, triglycerides, glycerin, squalane, hydrogenated lecithin	–
Physiogel AI cream/lotion	Aqua, olea europaea, glycerin, pentylene glycol, palm glycerides, olus, hydrogenated lecithin, palmitamide MEA, squalance, betaine, palmitamide MEA, sarcosine, acetamide MEA, hydroxyethyl-cellulose, sodium carbomer, carbomer, xanthan gum	PEA, a physiological complex with anti-oxidant properties DMS® (Derma Membrane Structure)
Atogla	Aqua, mineral oil, glycerin, *Borage officinalis* seed oil, *Triticum vulgare* (wheat) germ oil, steareth-10 allyl ether/acrylates copolymer, stearic acid, laureth-23, steareth-2, ceteth-20, *Aloe barbadensis*, ceramide, *Butyrospermum parkii* (Shea) seed butter, microcrystalline wax, triethanolamine, diazolidinyl urea, pentaerythrityl tetra-di-t-butyl hydroxyhydrocinnamate, tris (tetramethylhydroxy piperidinol) citrate, disodium EDTA, methylchlorosothiazolinone, methylisothiazolinone, perfume	0.5% w/w gamma linolenic acid (from borage oil), ceramide (Uniblend II), 10% w/w aloe vera gel, 2% w/w wheat germ oil

Vitamin E acetate in cream |
Cetaphil RestoraDerm	Water, glycerin, caprylic/capric triglyceride, *Helianthus annuus* (sunflower) seed oil, pentylene glycol, shea butter, sorbitol, cyclopentasiloxane, cetearyl alcohol, behenyl alcohol, glyceryl stearate, tocopheryl acetate, hydroxypalmitoyl sphinganine, niacinamide, allantoin, panthenol, arginine, disodium ethylene dicocamide PEG-15 disulfate, glyceryl stearate citrate, sodium PCA, ceteareth-20, sodium polyacrylate, caprylyl glycol, citric acid, dimethiconol, disodium EDTA, sodium hyaluronate, cetyl alcohol	Filaggrin breakdown components (arginine and sodium PCA) and ceramides
Atopiclair	Hyaluronic acid, shea butter, *Vitis vinifera* (grapevine), telmesteine, vitamin C and E, ethylhexyl palmitate, pentylene glycol, arachidyl alcohol, behenyl alcohol, arachidyl glucoside, glyceryl stearate, butylene glycol, caprylol glycine, tocopheryl acetate, carbomer, ethylhexyl glycerine, piroctone olamine, sodium hydroxide and allantoin	Glycyrrhetinic acid
Rebask cream	Cholesterol, squalene, sodium hyaluronate, white soft paraffin, glycerin and dimethicone	Ceramide dominant
Oilatum cream	Light liquid paraffin, white soft paraffin	–
Oilatum lotion	Light liquid paraffin, white soft paraffin, providone K29, shea butter, glycerin	–
Oilatum emollient	Light liquid paraffin-63.4% w/w, isopropyl plamitate, isopropyl alcohol	–
Oilatum bar	Mineral oil, sodium palmate, glycerin, corn oil	–
Emoderm cream	White soft paraffin	–

MEA, monoethanolamine; PEA, palmitoylethanolamine; EDTA, ethylenediaminetetraacetic acid; PEG, polyethylene glycol; PCA, pyrrolidone carboxylic acid.

parameters, quality of life, and patient acceptability are needed. The ideal skin barrier therapeutic agent has not yet been delineated.[3]

CONCLUSION

Realistically, AD is a complex disease whose effective management should be individualized and holistic. It should encompass an assessment of severity and impact on quality of life, treatment of the inflamed epidermal skin barrier, recognition and treatment of infection, and assessment and management of environmental and allergic triggers. Patient and family education that seeks to maximize understanding and compliance with treatment is also important in all children with AD.[3] The application of moisturizers should be an integral part of the treatment of patients with AD as there is strong evidence that their use can reduce disease severity and the need for pharmacologic intervention (strength of recommendation-A and level of evidence-I).[6] The choice of moisturizing agent is highly dependent on individual preference. The ideal agent should be safe, effective, inexpensive, and free of additives, fragrances, perfumes, and other potentially sensitizing agents. Therefore, it may be a matter of trial and error to find the most suitable formulation for an individual. Today, the best product for an individual may be the one they prefer because they will use it regularly and it will, therefore, be effective.

REFERENCES

1. Gelmetti C, Wollenberg A. Atopic dermatitis--all you can do from the outside. Br J Dermatol. 2014;170 Suppl 1:19-24.
2. Oranje AP. Proactive Therapy and Emollient Therapy in Atopic Dermatitis. Current Treatment Options in Allergy. 2014;1:365-73.
3. Hon KL, Leung AK, Barankin B. Barrier repair therapy in atopic dermatitis: an overview. Am J Clin Dermatol. 2013;14(5):389-99.
4. Wolf R, Parish LC. Barrier-repair prescription moisturizers: do we really need them? Facts and controversies. Clin Dermatol. 2013;31(6):787-91.
5. Wolf R, Wolf D. Abnormal epidermal barrier in the pathogenesis of atopic dermatitis. Clin Dermatol. 2012;30(3):329-34.
6. Eichenfield LF, Tom WL, Berger TG, et al. Guidelines of care for the management of atopic dermatitis: section 2. Management and treatment of atopic dermatitis with topical therapies. J Am Acad Dermatol. 2014;71(1):116-32.
7. Lodén M. The skin barrier and use of moisturizers in atopic dermatitis. Clin Dermatol. 2003;21(2):145-57.

CHAPTER 6

Moisturizers in Acne

Rashmi Sarkar, Shilpa Garg

INTRODUCTION

Increased sebum production is one of the etiopathological causes of acne and patients with acne generally complain of oily skin. As physicians, we usually advise our acne patients to keep the skin dry by washing the face twice a day and by avoiding the use of moisturizing agents. However, some recent evidence has shown that acne by itself and certain medications prescribed for its treatment may cause dysfunction of epidermal barrier with increase in transepidermal water loss (TEWL) and lead to symptoms of dryness, redness, subjective irritation, pruritus, increased skin sensitivity and discomfort to the patient. This can lead to nonadherence with treatment and treatment failure. Therefore, management of acne by physicians has now evolved and expanded beyond just prescribing drugs and focuses on four primary fundamental goals: (1) cleansing, (2) medicating, (3) moisturizing, and (4) photoprotection.[1] Hence, it has now become important for physicians to involve themselves in the holistic management of acne including proper skin care and product selection.

CAUSES OF EPIDERMAL BARRIER DYSFUNCTION IN ACNE VULGARIS

Acne by itself and certain topical agents used for acne therapy such as benzoyl peroxide, retinoids, alcohol-based antibiotic preparations and salicylic acid can lead to skin dryness and irritation, resulting in poor compliance with therapy and compromised efficacy. The various factors which result in epidermal barrier dysfunction and lead to an increase in TEWL in patients with acne are as follows:
- *Epidermal barrier impairment innate to acne vulgaris*: There is some evidence to suggest that impairment of stratum corneum permeability barrier is innate to acne vulgaris.[2] Yamamoto, et al. reported that patients with acne had higher levels of sebum secretion and TEWL along with decreased stratum corneum conductance and hydration, suggesting an innate impairment of stratum corneum permeability barrier.[3] Also patients with acne vulgaris had markedly diminished levels of free sphingosine, linoleic acid and total ceramides in stratum corneum, causing deficiency of the intercellular lipid

membrane, leading to increased TEWL and stratum corneum permeability barrier dysfunction.[4] The magnitude of stratum corneum permeability barrier impairment was found to correlate directly with the severity of acne vulgaris.[3] A study found that the mean percentage of total ceramides present in the polar lipid fraction of stratum corneum from acne patients was significantly lower as compared to matched controls without acne. Stratum corneum is primarily composed of ceramides, free fatty acids, and cholesterol, which play a role in maintaining its barrier function by restricting water movement and penetration. It is hypothesized that ceramide deficiency resulting in impaired skin barrier can promote follicular hyperkeratosis leading to comedone formation.

- *Medication-induced epidermal changes*: Certain medications which are used for treatment of acne vulgaris can induce changes in the stratum corneum permeability barrier. These are:
  o Benzoyl peroxide: Benzoyl peroxide has been shown to adversely affect the epidermal barrier function by causing impairment in the antioxidant barrier and stratum corneum permeability barrier.[2] A study by Weber, et al. showed an increase in TEWL by 1.8-fold by 10% formulation of benzoyl peroxide along with reduced cutaneous levels of vitamin E.[5] In a study by Feldman, et al., an internet-based survey was carried out in 200 acne patients to find the self-reported irritation and its impact of using fixed combination of clindamycin and 5% benzoyl peroxide. Bothersome side effects reported by patients were: dry skin (55%), flaky/peeling skin (45%), irritated skin (44%), itchy skin (39%) and redness (37%). Due to these side effects, 33% patients used the product only as a spot treatment, 28% patients used it only when breakouts seemed worse, 32% used it less often than recommended, 32% stopped using it from time to time, 28% changed to a different medication and 10% patients stopped using the product. Forty one percent patients were using moisturizers to alleviate dryness and redness.[6]
  o Retinoids: Retinoids cause accelerated epidermal cell turnover with thickening of lower epidermis and thinning of stratum corneum with microfissure formation. This together with an increased TEWL leads to compromised stratum corneum barrier function. This manifests as "retinoid dermatitis" characterized by erythema, fine scaling, desquamation and irritation, which usually happens within the initial 1–3 weeks of therapy. This is often mild and transient and resolve after a few weeks. Oral isotretinoin induced xerotic and desquamative cutaneous changes due to stratum corneum dyscohesion are not induced by changes in epidermal surface lipids due to the sebosuppressive effects and altered sebum lipid content caused by oral retinoids. These changes are greater in magnitude with oral than with topical retinoid therapy. Mildly visible but tolerable retinoid dermatitis can be mitigated with proper skin care. In case of severe retinoid dermatitis, retinoid should be temporarily discontinued. This should be coupled with proper adjunctive skin care, use of vehicle known to be well tolerated, stopping the retinoid for 5–7 days and then restarting with a reduced frequency of application (i.e. every other night

instead of every night) for the first few weeks, and using a topical retinoid with a track record of low irritation potential and comparable efficacy. In a study, 50 women were treated for facial photoaging with tretinoin cream 0.025%. It was observed that use of moisturizer 2 weeks prior and during tretinoin treatment prevented an increase in TEWL.[3] A randomized, investigator/evaluator-blinded, split face study of 174 healthy subjects was conducted, in which tretinoin cream 0.05% was applied once daily on the whole face and a moisturizer with sun-protection factor (SPF) 30 was applied to one side of the face. Skin irritation was experienced by approximately 85% of the subjects on both sides of their face, but it was predominantly milder on the side treated with moisturizer. In a 4-week, randomized, investigator-blinded, split face study of 30 healthy volunteers, adapalene gel was applied to the whole face and a moisturizing lotion was applied to only one side of the face once daily. Better tolerance was reported by the subjects and investigators on the side of moisturizing lotion with adapalene at each visit with significant difference reported by the subjects during the first 2 weeks (p = 0.039 and 0.013, respectively). The global worst score (average of worst scores for erythema, desquamation, dryness, stinging/burning and pruritus) was also significantly lower for the side of moisturizing lotion with adapalene as compared to the side of adapalene gel alone (0.43 ± 0.34 vs. 0.59 ± 0.44, p = 0.032). This study concluded that the adjunctive usage of a moisturizer improves the tolerance and adherence to adapalene gel.[7] The local tolerance of adapalene is more among Asians than Caucasians, as Asian skin is believed to be more susceptible than Caucasian skin. In a study, 30 patients on either oral isotretinoin or topical tretinoin were treated with twice daily application of a moisturizing agent involving one side of the face. Patients reported significant improvement in their skin dryness, roughness and desquamation. There was also improvement in skin properties and discomfort.[8]

So the authors suggest that it is important to first inform the patients regarding the possibility of irritation with these agents and advise them to start application on alternate nights, initiate therapy with low-strength preparations, gentle application of topical agent on skin and to wash the topical retinoids in the morning. If, however, in spite of this the patient continues to have skin irritation, then moisturizer should be prescribed concomitantly in order to alleviate skin irritation and dryness, enhance efficacy, increase compliance with treatment and improve skin comfort. If the problem still does not get solved, then it is advisable to switch to alternative treatment regimens.

- Moisturizers may also need to be prescribed in individuals with acne who have co-existent atopic dermatitis, sensitive skin or are living in climatic conditions with severe winters or low humidity as all these can cause impairment of the epidermal barrier and associated skin sensitivity. The moisturizer may also assist in preventing residual hyperpigmentation resulting from skin irritation and inflammation, especially in those with darker skin type. Apart from these, there is some evidence that moisturizers can independently contribute in improving the signs and symptoms of acne.[1]

> **Box 1: Indications of moisturizers in patients with acne**
> - To combat skin irritation caused by various topical antiacne therapy
> - To combat excessive dryness of skin caused by oral isotretinoin therapy for acne
> - Patients with acne and atopic dermatitis
> - Patients with acne and sensitive skin
> - Patients with acne living in areas with extreme winters which leads to seasonal skin dryness.

INDICATIONS OF MOISTURIZERS IN PATIENTS WITH ACNE

The patients of acne in whom application of moisturizing agents may be required and recommended is mentioned in Box 1.

CONSTITUENTS OF VARIOUS MOISTURIZERS USED FOR ACNE

Dermatologist-directed skin care beyond the selection of prescription therapies is very important as it:
- Makes a patient feel a sense of strong professional interest taken by the doctor in managing their acne
- Obviates the questions and confusion regarding the general skin care including what products to use and how to integrate them with prescribed topical medication. These questions are in the patients' mind but often are not asked by them
- Reduces the likelihood of self-selection of skin care and non-prescription products by the patient which can induce skin irritation that can sabotage the acne therapy prescribed by the dermatologist.

General skin care advice by a dermatologist should focus on selection of a gentle cleanser, moisturizer as well as photoprotectant formulation.

An ideal moisturizer should be non-comedogenic and should not worsen acne, should have no sensitization or irritation potential, diminish facial shine and skin oiliness, decrease the TEWL, increase the skin hydration, should be cosmetically acceptable and incorporate a broad-spectrum photoprotection.

In a study by Chularojanamontri et al. 52 products of moisturizers that are available online and over-the-counter and which claim to be suitable for acne, blemishes, and pimples were selected and their ingredients and properties were identified.[9] The ingredients in the product had occlusive, humectants, emollient, anti-inflammatory and oil reducing properties (Table 1). Other than occlusive, humectant and emollient effects, anti-inflammatory properties were present in 92% (48/52) of the products. More than 50% of the products contained dimethicone and/or glycerin for their moisturizing effect. Other commonly used ingredients were botanical anti-inflammatories like aloe vera and witch hazel. Due to their drawbacks for acne-prone skin, ingredients like petrolatum, lanolin, and mineral oil, were only occasionally added. A randomized controlled study by Park et al. showed that addition of evening primrose oil containing gamma-linolenic acid lead to improvement in the barrier function of lipids and prevents oral isotretinoin-induced adverse effects without any complications in patients taking oral isotretinoin. However, the statistical correlation between the evening primrose oil and xerotic cheilitis was found to be relatively weak in this study.

Table 1: Active ingredients and properties of moisturizers for acne in various products available online and over-the-counter

Properties	Ingredients
Occlusive	Beeswax, caprylic/capric triglyceride, cetyl alcohol, cocoa butter, cyclomethicone, dimethicone, glyceryl stearate, grape seed oil, lanolin (wool alcohol), lecithin
Humectant	Betaine, butylene glycol, cetearyl isononanoate, glycerin (glycerol), honey, hyaluronic acid, jojoba oil, lactic acid
Emollient	Almond oil, arachidyl alcohol, cetearyl alcohol, cholesterol, cyclomethicone, cyclopentasiloxane, decyl oleate, dimethicone, ethylhexyl palmitate, fatty acids, glyceryl stearate, isohexadecane, isopropyl myristate, lanolin (wool alcohol)
Anti-inflammatory	Aloe vera (*Aloe barbadensis*), beeswax, bisabolol, chamomile (*Matricaria recutita*), coconut oil, cucumber extract, glycyrrhetinic acid, green tea extract, *Hypericum perforatum* (St. John's wort), licochalcone A, benzoyl peroxide
Oil reducing	Licochalcone A

Evening primrose oil is a fatty acid found primarily in vegetable oils and improves skin hydration.

Silicone derivatives like dimethicone and cyclomethicone are usually used in oil-free facial moisturizers. The term "oil-free" implies that the substance does not contain either mineral or vegetable oil. Dimethicone is a non-comedogenic, non-acnegenic, hypoallergenic substance that is suitable for patients with acne and sensitive skin. It has occlusive and emollient properties and reduces TEWL without causing a greasy feel. Cyclomethicone is a thicker silicone with similar properties as dimethicone.

The use of lanolin is limited by its odor, expense and its propensity for causing allergic contact dermatitis. Though mineral oil (available in different grades) is lightweight, inexpensive, odorless and tasteless, it is not frequently used as it is comedogenic. However, it is considered that cosmetic grade mineral oil is non-comedogenic and industrial grade mineral oil is comedogenic.

Glycerin is the most effective humectant, but if used in high concentration it can cause a sticky feeling on skin. This can be decreased with addition of other humectants like hyaluronic acid and sodium pyrrolidone carboxylic acid (PCA). It is important to remember that use of humectants alone can increase the TEWL (e.g. glycerin which can increase TEWL by 29%). Hence, a humectant is generally combined with an occlusive agent when used as a moisturizer. In the study by Chularojanamontri L, et al., glycerin (humectant) and dimethicone (occlusive agent) were generally used in combination in the products analyzed.[9]

Jojoba oil is a wax ester and contains mixture of naturally-occurring esters, tocopherols, sterols, and other unsaponifiable matter. It is an excellent moisturizer for acne patients as it does not block skin pores, helps to restore the normal oil balance of the skin, and has anti-inflammatory and antibacterial properties. Jojoba oil is stable to oxidation and imparts photoprotection.[6]

Sesame oil is mainly composed of triglycerides of oleic acid, linoleic acid and a small percentage of saturated fats. It contains antioxidants and has oil pulling property. It has vitamin E, which imparts moisturizing and emollient properties.[6]

Almond oils are glycerides of oleic and linoleic acid, phytosterols, α-tocopherol and vitamin K. Upon topical application, fatty acids get metabolized in the skin and normalize the lipid layer and improve the water retention capability of the skin. α-tocopherol increases the water-binding ability of the skin and hence, improves the appearance of rough and damaged skin. Also it does not clog pores or leave the skin oily. Wheat germ oil is one of the richest sources of vitamin A, E, and D and has high content of lecithin and proteins. It helps to combat skin irritation, dryness and cracking.

Botanical extracts have anti-inflammatory properties and aloe vera, *Ginkgo biloba*, green tea, allantoin and licochalcone are commonly used ingredients in the current market. Aloe vera and witch hazel also possesses skin-soothing properties. The anti-inflammatory effect of aloe vera is due to the inhibition of cyclo-oxygenase in the arachidonic pathway. For moisturizing effect, the concentration of aloe vera should be at least 10%. Witch hazel is commonly used as an astringent in people who have oily skin. Hamamelis ointments, also known as witch hazel ointments, are used as acne cosmeceuticals.

Metals such as zinc, copper, selenium, aluminum, and strontium have anti-inflammatory properties and are used in cosmeceuticals. The anti-inflammatory response of zinc is because of its requirement by alkaline phosphatase in the adenosine monophosphate metabolism. Oral zinc has been shown to be effective in the treatment of acne due to its action on the inflammatory cells, especially granulocytes. Topical zinc may have a sebosuppressive effect due to its antiandrogen activity through inhibition of 5α-reductase. In a double-blind, randomized trial, 14 subjects applied a 4% erythromycin plus 1.2% zinc topical formulation on half of their foreheads, and a 4% erythromycin lotion on the other half of their foreheads twice daily for 3 months. There was significant reduction in subjects' casual level of sebum, sebum excretion rates, and total area of lipid spots on the side treated with 4% erythromycin plus 1.2% zinc topical formulation.

Moisturizers may also incorporate certain sebum absorbant ingredients such as silica microbeads, corn starch, kaolin, talc and bentonite which help in oil control by absorption of skin surface sebum to reduce facial shine. Addition of such ingredients is helpful for oily skin, but are not problematic for non-oily skin and does not cause dryness in them. The reduction of both sebum production and facial shine is important in the management of psychosocial morbidities of acne patients as facial shine can be emotionally disconcerting.

Pseudo-ceramide-5 (5 N-2-hydroxyhexadecanoyl sphinganine) gets incorporated as physiological lipids in stratum corneum through likely conversion to endogenous ceramide and helps to maintain barrier integrity and function. Phytosphingosine is a ceramide sphingolipid ingredient which has both antimicrobial activity against *Propionibacterium acnes* and anti-inflammatory action.

Ingredient like dipotassium glycyrrhizate which is derived from licorice root has anti-inflammatory properties by inhibiting superoxide formation, cyclo-oxygenase activity and breakdown of cortisol in skin. In acne vulgaris, induction of inflammatory reactions occurs via the cyclo-oxygenase-2 (COX-2) and prostaglandin E2 (PGE2) pathway. Licorice derivatives help in counteracting this inflammatory cascade by suppressing the inflammatory responses of the COX-2 and PGE2 pathway.

Ingredients like Span 60 and Tween 20 are added as emulsifying agents. Carbopol 940 is added as a gelling agent. Butylated hydroxytoluene has antioxidant properties and disodium ethylenediaminetetraacetic acid (EDTA) is used as a chelating agent. Methyl paraben and propyl paraben are used as preservatives.[6]

CONCLUSION

Management of patients with acne has now expanded beyond medical prescription of drugs and a holistic management should incorporate dermatologist-selected skin care. Prescribing a medication for acne without reviewing a patient's skin care regimen may lead to poor compliance, intolerable side effects, treatment failure and patient and physician frustration. It is important to strike a delicate balance between maintaining the skin barrier while controlling oil and shine in the skin. Hence, the treating physicians must be aware of the ingredients and properties of moisturizers which are suitable for use in acne patients. Physicians should consider including use of moisturizers (Table 2) if indicated from both scientific and patient preference point of view in patients affected by acne, especially those undergoing treatment with topical therapy for acne vulgaris.

Table 2: Moisturizers available in India for acne

Name of the product	Ingredients
Acnemoist cream	• Pentavitin 1% w/w • Jojoba ester 3% w/w • Octyl methoxy cinnamate (OMC) 5% • MBBT 4%
SebaMed clear face care gel for acne prone skin Free from oils and emulsifiers	Aqua, *Aloe barbadensis* leaf juice, propylene glycol, glycerine, sorbitol, panthenol, sodium hyaluronate, allantoin, sodium carbomer, sodium citrate, phenoxyethanol
Acrofy	Purified water, glycerin, propylene glycol, niacinamide, aqua-butylene glycol-PEG-60 almond glycerides-caprylyl glycol-glycerin-carbomer-nordihydroguaiaretic acid-oleanolic acid, Imperata cylindrical-aqua-glycerin-PEG 8-carbomer, polyamide 5, shea butter, glyceryl stearate, PEG 100 stearate, cetyl alcohol, cyclomethicone and dimethicone copolyol, ethylhexyl palmitate-sorbitan oleate-sorbitan laurate-myristyl phosphor-malate, sodium acrylates copolymer lecithin, sodium gluconate and lactate derivative, stearyl alcohol, sorbitan monostearate, citric acid, propyl paraben, butylated hydroxytoluene, disodium edentate, methyl paraben, ascorbyl palmitate
Cetaphil dermacontrol moisturizing SPF30+	• Glycerin • Panthenol • Pentylene glycol • Zinc gluconate • Silica • Polymethyl methacrylate

Continued

Continued

Name of the product	Ingredients
Table 2: Moisturizers available in India for acne	
	• Avobenzone 3% • Octisalate 5% • Octocrylane 5% • Hydroxypalmitoyl sphinganine • Allantoin • Glycyrrhetinic acid • Isopropyl lauryl sarcosinate • Dimethicone • Dimethiconol • Caprylyl glycol
Aveeno DML lotion (Daily moisturizing lotion)	Aqua, glycerin, distearyldimonium chloride, petrolatum, isopropyl palmitate, cetyl alcohol, dimethicone, *Avena sativa* (oat) kernel flour, benzyl alcohol, sodium chloride
Aveeno SRL lotion (Skin relief moisturizing lotion)	Aqua, glycerin, distearyldimonium chloride, petrolatum, isopropyl palmitate, cetyl alcohol, dimethicone, *Avena sativa* (oat) kernel flour, *A. sativa* (oat) kernel oil, benzyl alcohol, Butyrospermum parkii (shea butter) extract, Steareth-20+ *A. sativa* (oat) kernel extract, sodium chloride
Physiogel lotion (hypoallergenic)	Phospholipids, triglycerides, squalene, cholestrol, ceramides
Physiogel cream (hypoallergenic)	Phospholipids, triglycerides, squalene, cholestrol, ceramides

PEG, polyethylene glycol; MBBT, methylene bis-benzotriazolyl tetramethylbutylphenol.

REFERENCES

1. Del Rosso JQ, Gold M, Rueda MJ, et al. Efficacy, safety, and subject satisfaction of a specified skin care regimen to cleanse, medicate, moisturize, and protect the skin of patients under treatment for acne vulgaris. J Clin Aesthet Dermatol. 2015;8(1):22-30.
2. Del Rosso JQ. The role of skin care as an integral component in the management of acne vulgaris: part 1: the importance of cleanser and moisturizer ingredients, design, and product selection. J Clin Aesthet Dermatol. 2013;6(12):19-27.
3. Yamamoto A, Takenouchi K, Ito M. Impaired water barrier function in acne vulgaris. Arch Dermatol Res. 1995;287(2):214-8.
4. Thiboutot D, Del Rosso JQ. Acne vulgaris and the epidermal barrier: is acne vulgaris associated with inherent epidermal abnormalities that cause impairment of barrier functions? Do any topical acne therapies alter the structural and/or functional integrity of the epidermal barrier? J Clin Aesthet Dermatol. 2013;6(2):18-24.
5. Weber SU, Thiele JJ, Han N, et al. Topical tocotrienol supplementation inhibits lipid peroxidation but fails to mitigate increased transepidermal water loss after benzoyl peroxide treatment of human skin. Free Radical Biology Medicine. 2003;34:170-6.
6. Thakur NK, Bharti P, Mahant S, et al. Formulation and Characterization of Benzoyl Peroxide Gellified Emulsions. Sci Pharm. 2012;80(4):1045-60.
7. Matsunaga K, Leow YH, Chan R, et al. Adjunctive usage of a non-comedogenic moisturizer with adapalene gel 0.1% improves local tolerance: a randomized, investigator-blinded, split-face study in healthy Asian subjects. Journal of Dermatological Treatment. 2013; 24(4):278-82.
8. Laquieze S, Czernielewski J, Rueda MJ. Beneficial effect of a moisturizing cream as adjunctive treatment to oral isotretinoin or topical tretinoin in the management of acne. J Drugs Dermatol. 2006;5(10):985-90.
9. Chularojanamontri L, Tuchinda P, Kulthanan K, et al. Moisturizers for acne. What are their constituents? J Clin Aesthet Dermatol. 2014;7(5):36-44.

CHAPTER 7

Moisturizers in Rosacea and Sensitive Skin

Surabhi Sinha

INTRODUCTION

Rosacea patients are often known to possess sensitive or hyperirritable skin. Similarly, patients with "sensitive skin" may complain of burning/stinging/tingling or itching sensations after application of normally innocuous toiletries or cosmetics. Thus, such patients need an appropriate skin care regime consisting of cleansing, moisturizing and sun protection with agents that would not contain/contain only minimal amounts of potentially "irritating" ingredients. Here, we seek to delve on the important topic of moisturizers for such patients.

ROSACEA

Rosacea is a common chronic dermatosis. It is characterized, alone or in combination, by central facial erythema, symmetric flushing, stinging, inflammatory lesions, papules and pustules, telangiectases, and phymatous changes. Due to the variation in the signs and symptoms, the therapy too has to be tailored to each specific patient.

Besides the objective signs, the subjective sensation of stinging, burning, tingling, itching, tightness as well as hyperirritability of the skin are equally discomforting to the patient. These symptoms are indicative of inherent "sensitive skin".[1] Both male and female patients commonly report that their skin is often very sensitive to many skin care and personal care products. In a study by Torok, female patients reported skin sensitivity most commonly to astringents and toners, soap and exfoliating agents.[2] Male patients reported skin sensitivity to soap, followed by cologne and shaving lotion.[2]

Rosacea has five major subtypes: (1) Erythematotelangiectatic rosacea (ETR), (2) papulopustular rosacea (PPR), (3) phymatous rosacea, (4) granulomatous rosacea and (5) ocular rosacea. The first two are the major subtypes with ETR: PPR = 7:3 approximately.

Dryness and tightness of the skin are frequent in rosacea; hence the utility of moisturizers is justified. However, a growing body of evidence suggests that moisturizer use can play a more important adjunctive role in improving skin homeostasis and deficient stratum corneum (SC) barrier function, and thus in the holistic treatment of rosacea.

SENSITIVE SKIN

Sensitive skin can be defined as abnormal subclinical sensory responses to drugs, cosmetics and toiletries in the absence of visible signs of irritation.[3] The complaints commonly associated include itching, burning, stinging and tightness of the skin. Triggers include cosmetics, drugs and toiletries, plus environmental factors like ultraviolet light, heat, cold and wind. Different synonyms have been used to describe this entity, including reactive, hyper-reactive, intolerant and irritable skin. Due to the absence of specific clinical signs, no clear consensual definition has yet been accepted. It is often a self-diagnosed and self-declared condition, without evident clinical traits, and is, thus, tough to quantify and still tougher to manage!

It usually concerns the face because of its denser nervous network and its great exposure to cosmetic or physical triggering factors. Nevertheless, it is not limited to the face, and sensitive skin may arise on hands or the scalp too.[4] Visible signs such as erythema or scaling are usually not present. Patients may report feeling dryness or tightness several washing/moisturizing cycles before observable signs of dryness appear.

Sensitive skin may occur in isolation or along with specific skin diagnoses such as atopic dermatitis, rosacea, acute contact eczema, etc. The work-up and management should include a complete 2-week discontinuation of any topical application, except for synthetic detergent (syndet) bar, clinical examination for underlying dermatoses (rosacea, atopic dermatitis, psoriasis, etc.), a test battery (patch, photopatch, lactic acid stinging test, contact urticaria) and a progressive reintroduction of the cosmetics and skin care products according to a specific protocol.

Suitable cleansers and therapeutic moisturizers are of benefit as adjuncts to alleviate dryness, restore skin barrier function and reduce susceptibility to irritation in these patients.

MOISTURIZERS

A "moisturizer" is an agent designed to make the SC soft and more pliant by increasing the hydration of dry skin thus, resulting in smoother, suppler and healthier looking skin.[5]

The three basic types of moisturizers are:
1. *Occlusives*: Occlusives form a layer on the skin that is poorly permeated by water. They are especially effective when applied to already dampened skin. Thus, they reduce transepidermal water loss (TEWL). They are the most common type of moisturizers used. Petrolatum followed by dimethicone (silicone derivative) are the two most common occlusives used. Both are hypoallergenic, non-comedogenic and non-acnegenic. However, occlusives have the limitations of odor, greasy feel and potential allergenicity.
   Examples: *Petrolatum* (prototype), silicone derivatives, mineral oil, caprylic/capric triglyceride, lanolin, cetyl alcohol, stearyl alcohol.
2. *Humectants*: Humectants increase SC hydration by attracting and holding water in the SC (either from dermis or from the environment).
   Examples: Glycerin (prototype), propylene glycol, ammonium lactate, potassium lactate, sodium lactate, sodium pyrrolidone carboxylic acid (PCA),

hyaluronic acid, sorbitol, urea, polyglyceryl methacrylate, and alpha-hydroxy acids (AHAs)—lactic acid, glycolic acid, tartaric acid.

Urea and AHAs are keratolytic, and thus may cause irritation and stinging on the skin of patients with rosacea and sensitive skin.

3. *Emollients*: Emollients are materials designed to make the skin feel and appear smooth by filling the spaces between the skin flakes with droplets of oil. Some may have additional occlusive properties.

Examples: Mineral oil, cholesterol, squalene, glycerol stearate, soy sterol, lanolin, sunflower seed oil.

The standard components in a conventional oil-in-water over-the-counter (OTC) facial moisturizer include approximately 80% water, 5% humectants, 4% occlusives/emollients, 6% emulsifiers, 2% silicate, 0.3% thickeners, 0.4% preservatives and 0.2% fragrance.[6] However, this is by no means uniform. In addition, nowadays there are further advancements available:

- The ability to deposit specific lipids within the SC
- The ability to deposit specific humectants to enhance SC hydration
- The ability to provide occlusivity to reduce TEWL
- Better cosmetic acceptability and better "feel" and "elegance" of products
- Avoidance of ingredients with high propensity of allergic/irritant contact reactions.

Addition of physiologic lipids and humectants or occlusive would benefit patients with rosacea or sensitive skin. However, they should be present in the correct ratios to be effective and free from adverse effects.

As previously mentioned, the basic function of a moisturizer is to provide hydration to the SC. This can be achieved by direct and indirect mechanisms. Direct mechanism is via occlusion and consequent decrease of TEWL (e.g., petrolatum), but the total improvement in skin hydration may not be very significant.

Indirect mechanisms include the use of humectants and the incorporation of physiologic lipids that are actively packaged into lamellar bodies in the stratum granulosum and deposited in the upper SC. This is a slower mechanism but the reparative effects on the SC permeability barrier are more prolonged.

POTENTIAL ADVERSE EFFECTS OF MOISTURIZER INGREDIENTS

Petrolatum is the prototype and the most effective occlusive (98% reduction of SC water loss) as it diffuses into the intercellular lipid bilayer of the skin. However, this may also interfere with the SC barrier recovery, and hence petrolatum is not the best choice for patients with impaired SC permeability barrier such as rosacea and sensitive skin. Similarly, propylene glycol (PEG) and PCA may rarely produce irritant reactions in patients with sensitive skin and rosacea. PEG is also susceptible to oxidation and may release free radical species, hence may not be ideal in rosacea patients. AHAs, urea, alcohol, acetone and menthol should also be avoided in view of potential irritation. Lanolin can cause allergic and irritant reactions. Fragrances too should be avoided in products meant to be applied to sensitive skin.

MOISTURIZERS IN ROSACEA AND SENSITIVE SKIN

The innate disturbance of the SC permeability barrier correlates with increased centrofacial TEWL which in turn appears to account for the skin sensitivity in patients with rosacea.[7-9] Thus, these patients may benefit immensely from an appropriate skin care regime which includes cleansing, sun protection and especially moisturizing. However, it is difficult for rosacea patients to discern which products and ingredients will benefit their skin and which may lead to an exacerbation of their disease. Thus, as dermatologists it is imperative for us to know the ingredients of the OTC and prescription products likely to be used by patients so as to guide them (Tables 1 and 2). Products that would benefit the patients would increase skin hydration, mitigate damage to SC proteins, limit damage and stripping of SC lipids, would not contain additives that could augment cutaneous irritation and would optimally deposit lipids, humectants, and cosmetically acceptable occlusive agents that could expedite SC repair.[8,10-15]

Levin and Miller also postulated that "priming" the skin in rosacea patients with an acute flare with a mild OTC cleanser and moisturizer for 3-5 days (with or without oral therapy according to clinical severity) before starting topical therapy would serve to diminish the hyperirritable state of their skin and may increase tolerance to further topical medical treatment.[16]

Del Rosso conducted a split face study on the use of moisturizers for topical therapy of rosacea. The author prescribed 15% azelaic acid gel with/without a designated moisturizer on each half of the face in 102 adult patients with PPR.[17] Itching was found the most prevalent symptom and burning was the most frequently occurring symptom. The author found a significantly greater overall reduction on the side with the moisturizer as compared to the other side without the moisturizer being used ($p = 0.015$). Thus, the author concluded that the inclusion of a moisturizer improves rosacea symptom relief.

In another controlled study by Draelos, et al., a 2% niacinamide (Vitamin B3)-containing moisturizer was shown to improve facial skin hydration in patients with rosacea.[18] It was also associated with reduction in erythema and inflammatory lesions as well as symptoms of dryness and scaling. The authors hypothesized that an improved SC barrier should be more resistant to penetration by noxious stimuli, and hence could improve the hyperirritability of the skin in rosacea patients.

Long-term steroid application is a common triggering factor for rosacea. Most steroid creams are drying and emollient-based moisturizers are, thus a useful adjunct to the therapeutic regime.

Regarding cosmetic use, cosmetic foundations should be lightweight, with an integrated broad-spectrum sunscreen preferably. Heavy cosmetics that are hard to remove should be avoided. Astringents, toners, abrasives and sensory stimulants (like camphor, menthol) should be avoided. Finally, green-tinted makeup and sunscreen can be used to disguise reddened areas of the face in rosacea. A handful of tinted moisturizers, are available now (Table 2). Patients can also be instructed to wait for 15-30 minutes after cleansing to allow drying of the skin (as many skin care products tend to be most irritating when applied to wet skin, presumably due to greater permeability of wet skin).

Table 1: Common chemical ingredients used in moisturizers

Chemical compound	Derived from	Function	Used in	Remarks
Glycerin	Natural	Humectant	Moisturizers	–
Petrolatum	Natural	Occlusive, emollient	Moisturizers	–
Ceramides 1-9	One of three lipids of stratum corneum	Physiologic lipid →Decrease TEWL	Moisturizers	Especially for sensitive skin and atopic dermatitis
Cholesterol	One of three lipids of stratum corneum	Emollient, skin conditioner, thickening agent, non-ionic emulsion stabilizer	Moisturizers	–
Cetearyl alcohol	Cetyl alcohol + stearyl alcohol (natural fatty alcohols in coconut oil)	Foam booster, viscosity enhancer, emulsion stabilizer, emollient	Moisturizers, hair conditioners	–
Ceteareth 20	Cetearyl alcohol + ethylene oxide	Emollient, emulsifier	Cosmetics, moisturizers, sunscreens, cleansers	Ethylene oxide and 1,4 dioxane—potential carcinogens—safety concerns
Behentrimonium methosulfate (BTMS) (usually used with cetearyl alcohol to boost effects)	Quaternary ammonium compound, from rapeseed oil	Cationic emulsifier, slippery feel	Lotions, shampoos, conditioners	Most promising hair detangler ever, allergic reactions known, may benefit rosacea patients as cationic so can bind to negatively charged keratin→persist after washing →longer moisturization
Capric/caprylic triglyceride	Oily liquid from coconut oil	Emollient, occlusive, slippery feel, promotes dispersion of pigment in colored cosmetics	Cosmetics, moisturizers, sunscreens	–
Simethicone/dimethicone	Silicon-based polymers	Occlusive, antifoaming, skin protectant, slippery feel, anti-inflammatory	Most skin care products—very safe compound	Decreases redness of rosacea, hence used with more irritating inorganic sunscreen agents

Continued

Continued

Table 1: Common chemical ingredients used in moisturizers

Chemical compound	Derived from	Function	Used in	Remarks
Hyaluronic acid	Natural polysaccharide	Humectant (holds 1,000 times water)	Anti-aging moisturizers	–
Carbomer	Made from acrylic acid	Emulsifier, holds water and swells	Moisturizers, cosmetics	–
Xanthum gum	Polysaccharide made by fermentation of sucrose by Xanthomonas campestris	Holds water and swells, smooth glide, thickener in emulsions	Moisturizers	–
Aloe vera	Natural	Anti-inflammatory	Moisturizers	Improves redness and inflammatory lesions of rosacea
Phytosphingosine	Natural sphingolipid	Antibacterial, anti-inflammatory	Conditioners, moisturizers	–
Sodium lauroyl lactylate (SLL)	Natural, from sodium salt of lactic acid	Foaming, smooth glide, humectant	Cosmetics, cleansers, moisturizers	–
Methyl/propyl parabens	Paraben	Preservatives	Cosmetics, moisturizers	Allergic reactions known
Phenoxyethanol	Green tea, synthetic also	Preservative	Cosmetics, moisturizers	One of the least irritating preservatives
Disodium ethylenediamine-tetraacetic acid (EDTA)	Synthetic	Preservative, stabilizer, metal chelator	Rinse-off hair products, moisturizers	Chelates metals in hard water →negates adverse effects on hair and skin

Table 2: Moisturizers available in India for rosacea and sensitive skin

Name of moisturizer	Main ingredients	Remarks
Cetaphil daily facial moisturizer	Glycerin, cyclomethicone	–
Cetaphil RESTORADERM skin restoring moisturizer	Glycerin, sorbitol, caprylic/capric triglyceride, sun flower seed oil, shea butter, cyclopentasiloxane, cetearyl alcohol	–
Neutrogena oil-free moisturizing cream (combination skin)	Glycerin, dimethicone, petrolatum	–
Eucerin redness relief soothing night crème	Glycerin, dimethicone, licochalcone (licorice root extract)	Tinted
Eucerin redness relief daily perfecting lotion SPF 15	Licochalcone, sunscreens	Tinted
CeraVe moisturizing cream	Glycerin, ceteareth 20, capric/caprylic triglyceride, BTMS, ceramides, cholesterol	–
Rosaliac anti-redness moisturizer	Glycerin, dimethicone, niacinamide, shea butter, carbomer, xanthan gum, parabens	–
Aderma epitheliale AH repair cream	Hyaluronic acid, Rhealba® oat	–
Aderma sensiphase moisturizer	Rhealba® oat, vitamin E	–
Avene redness relief moisturizing protecting cream SPF 20	Glycerin, cyclomethicone, sunscreens, methyl paraben	–
Vanicream moisturizing skin cream	Petrolatum, cetearyl alcohol, propylene glycol, ceteareth 20, simethicone	–
Clinique redness solutions daily relief cream	Dimethicone, shea butter, cetearyl alcohol, green tea leaf extract	Tinted (green) to negate the redness
Physiogel lotion (hypoallergenic)	Phospholipids, triglycerides, squalene, cholestrol, ceramides	–
Physiogel cream (hypoallergenic)	Phospholipids, triglycerides, squalene, cholestrol, ceramides	–

The ingredients commonly used in moisturizers and cosmetics and the moisturizers available for sensitive skin and rosacea have been summarized in Tables 1 and 2.

REFERENCES

1. Kligman AM. Human models for characterizing "sensitive skin". Cosmet Dermatol. 2001;14:15-9.
2. Torok HM. Rosacea skin care. Cutis. 2000;66(Suppl.4):14-6.
3. Kligman AM, Sadiq I, Zhen Y, et al. Experimental studies on the nature of sensitive skin. Skin Res Technol 2006;12(4):217-22.

4. Saint-Martory C, Roguedas-Contios AM, Sibaud V, et al. Sensitive skin is not limited to the face. Br J Dermatol. 2008;158:130-3.
5. Loden M. The clinical benefit of moisturizers. J Eur Acad Dermatol Venereol. 2005;19(6): 672-88.
6. Rawlings AV, Canestrari DA, Dobkowski B. Moisturizer technology versus clinical performance. Dermatol Ther. 2004;17:49-56.
7. Crawford GH, Pelle MH, James WD. Rosacea: I. Etiology, pathogenesis and subtype classification. J Am Acad Dermatol. 2004;51(3):327-41.
8. Cheong WK. Gentle cleansing and moisturizing for patients with atopic dermatitis and sensitive skin. Am J Clin Dermatol 2009;10 Suppl 1:13-7.
9. Dirschka T, Tronnier H, Fölster-Holst R. Epithelial barrier function and atopic diathesis in rosacea and perioral dermatitis. Br J Dermatol. 2004;150(6):1136-41.
10. Loden M. Role of topical emollients and moisturizers in the treatment of dry skin barrier disorders. Am J Clin Dermatol 2003;4(11):771-88.
11. Lonne-Rahm SB, Fischer T, Berg M. Stinging and rosacea. Acta Derm Venereol. 1999;79(6):460-1.
12. Draelos ZD. Cosmetics in acne and rosacea. Semin Cutan Med Surg. 2001;20(3):209-14.
13. Buraczewska I, Berne B, Lindberg M, et al. Changes in skin barrier function following long-term treatment with moisturizers, a randomized controlled trial. Br J Dermatol. 2007;156(3):492-8.
14. Del Rosso JQ. The role of maintaining proper barrier function in the management of rosacea. Cosmet Dermatol. 2007;20:485-90.
15. Del Rosso JQ. Adjunctive skin care in the management of rosacea: cleansers, moisturizers and photoprotectants. Cutis. 2005;75:17-21.
16. Levin J, Miller R. A guide to the ingredients and potential benefits of over-the-counter cleansers and moisturizers for rosacea patients. J Clin Aesthet Dermatol. 2011;4(8):31-49.
17. Del Rosso JQ. The use of moisturizers as an integral component of topical therapy for rosacea: clinical results based on assessment of skin characteristics study. Cutis. 2009;84(2):72-6.
18. Draelos ZD, Ertel K, Berge C. Niacinamide-containing facial moisturizer improves skin barrier and benefits subjects with rosacea. Cutis. 2005;76(2):135-41.

CHAPTER 8

Moisturizers for Xerotic and Ichthyotic Skin

Sayantani Chakraborty, Joyeeta Chowdhury

INTRODUCTION

Dry skin, or xerosis, is a common problem that most people experience to varying degrees at some stage in life. This may be due to altered environmental factors (e.g., seasons, climate, excessive bathing, use of harsh skin cleansers), while in others, endogenous factors such as deficiencies in the skin's natural moisturizing factor (NMF), barrier lipid content, or moisture network may be involved.[1]

Stratum corneum (SC) is the primary barrier of the skin which is rich in cholesterol, free fatty acids, and ceramides (CERs). Many oily preparations have been used to maintain the fluidity of the skin (mineral oil, lanolin, cyclomethicone, etc.). Water from the SC gets evaporated very quickly leading to dehydration.

Moisturizers by hydrating the skin, make the SC softer. When moisturizers are applied to the skin, a thin film of humectant is formed which retains moisture and imparts better appearance to the skin. Biomimetic lipid containing formulations facilitate in normalizing the damaged skin.

Ceramides and moisturizers containing CERs are used to treat xerotic and eczematous skin and maintain the balance of lipids in the skin.

The word *moisturizer* is a generic term used to encompass a multitude of formulations like emollients and humectant that vary widely in their capacity to provide therapeutically desirable effects such as barrier repair, reduced transepidermal water loss (TEWL), or esthetic improvement of irritated skin. They are formulated to maintain the water content of the skin between 10 and 30% as water is important to maintain plasticity and barrier integrity of skin.

PATHOPHYSIOLOGY OF XEROSIS AND ICHTHYOTIC SKIN

The primary function of the epidermis is to produce the protective, semipermeable SC. The barrier function of the SC is provided by patterned lipid lamellae localized to the extracellular spaces between corneocytes.

Certain genetic defects in lipid metabolism or in the protein components of the SC produce scaly or ichthyotic skin with abnormal barrier lipid structure and function.

Corneocytes when normally shed are not visible on the skin surface; when this process is disturbed in any way, corneocytes collect in visible clumps (scales) that produce a rough texture and appearance.

Majority of the population experience xerosis or "dry skin" at some stage in their lives.

Causes of Xerosis

Exogenous

- Cooler climates
- Winter
- Dry, hot climates
- Excessive bathing
- Cleansers containing surfactants.

Endogenous

- Age
- Atopy
- Endocrine diseases
- Chronic illness and nutritional deficiency
- Internal malignancy
- Medication.

Three key deficiencies in the skin have been shown to contribute to xerosis:
1. Deficiency in moisture-binding substances collectively known as the NMF.[2,3]
2. Deficiencies in the skin barrier lipids, CERs.[4]
3. Deficiency of the skin's own moisture network mediated by the newly discovered aquaporin water channels.[5]

Ichthyosis is a group of inherited and acquired disorders which result due to biochemical alteration of SC that leads to defective corneodesmolysis and retention of scales in fish-like pattern. This, however, represents defects in a complex array of molecules like filaggrin, proteolytic and lipolytic enzymes, CERs and other lipid components. In ichthyosis vulgaris, there is a profound deficiency in filaggrin; in lamellar ichthyosis due to transglutaminase 1 deficiency, abnormal cornified envelope leads to impaired barrier function. In epidermolytic hyperkeratosis, the barrier defect, however, has been shown to be due to abnormal lamellar granule secretion and the resulting decrease in SC lipid lamellae. A scoring system has been formulated for dry skin (Box 1).

Box 1: A scoring system for dry skin for use in clinical settings	
0	Absent
1	Faint scaling, faint roughness and dull appearance
2	Small scales in combination with a few larger scales, slight roughness, whitish appearance
3	Small and larger scales uniformly distributed, definite roughness, possibly slight redness and possibly a few superficial cracks
4	Dominated by large scales, advanced roughness, redness present, eczematous changes and cracks

In many inflammatory skin diseases where overall epidermal differentiation is disturbed, there are likely secondary effects on corneocyte structure and NMF generation as well as on the composition and function of the intercellular lipids that ultimately result in scaling.

SKIN HYDRATION AND BARRIER FUNCTION

The skin shows a unique mechanism of protection of underlying tissue from infection, drying and desiccation, chemical and mechanical stress. While the SC provides an effective barrier to water loss, there is some normal movement of water through it into the surrounding atmosphere, which is known as transepidermal water loss or TEWL which is very low in healthy skin and shows an increase in conditions like atopic dermatitis (AD), eczema and psoriasis.

Recent advances in knowledge about skin hydration have led to the development of new formulations with ingredients that specifically address the deficiencies in the physiologic mechanisms underlying xerotic conditions.

The factors which play a key role in maintaining skin hydration are:

Natural moisturizing factor: A collection of humectant substances originating from the catabolism of filaggrin, were first described in 1959 by Jacobi.[6]

The role of NMF is to maintain adequate SC hydration, which in turn serves three major functions:
1. Maintain plasticity of the skin, protecting it from damage.
2. Allow hydrolytic enzymes to function in the process of desquamation.
3. Contribute to optimum SC barrier function.

Reductions in NMF levels have been correlated with various SC abnormalities that clinically appear as areas of dry skin with scaling, flaking, and sometimes fissuring and cracking the components of NMF are given in Box 2.

These conditions include AD, psoriasis, ichthyosis vulgaris, and xerosis. In AD and xerosis, NMF levels are reduced, while in psoriatic skin and ichthyosis, NMF is essentially absent.[6]

Pyrrolidone carboxylic acid (PCA), the most prevalent single component of NMF, which on topical application has been widely reported to alleviate the symptoms of dry skin.

Several other NMF components; for instance, urea and lactate have been used in moisturizing creams. Topical application of urea, or its precursor arginine, has been shown to correct urea deficits in AD and elderly patients. Urea is used as a 10% cream for the treatment of ichthyosis and hyperkeratotic skin disorders.

Box 2: Chemical composition of natural moisturizing factor found in the epidermis

- Free amino acids
- Pyrrolidone carboxylic acid
- Lactate
- Sugars
- Urea
- Chloride
- Sodium
- Potassium
- Ammonia, uric acid, glucosamine, creatine
- Calcium
- Magnesium
- Phosphate
- Citrate, formate

It has also been shown to stimulate the expression of several enzymes involved in CER synthesis and barrier formation as well as the aquaporin-3 (AQP3) water channel in human keratinocytes.[7]

L-lactic acid and D,L-lactic acid appear to work by stimulating the synthesis of CERs in the SC.

Lipids: The three main lipid groups in the SC are CERs, free fatty acids, and cholesterol. At least nine different classes of CERs (1 to 9) have been described in the human SC, and of the total lipid mass present in the human SC, approximately 50% consists of CERs, with 25% consisting of cholesterol and 15% of free fatty acids.[8]

Stratum corneum lipids are essential for maintaining skin barrier function and preventing TEWL. Of the SC intercellular lipids, CERs are the most effective at restoring barrier function and increasing skin hydration. Not only quantitative reduction, but also the qualitative alteration like type and size of the molecule may affect the barrier function. For example, levels of CERs containing an ester-linked fatty acid and sphingosine are significantly lower in AD skin compared with healthy skin, whereas levels of CERs containing an alpha-hydroxy fatty acid and sphingosine were significantly higher in AD skin compared with healthy skin.

Increased CER synthesis accompanying improved barrier function has been seen in numerous studies employing agents ranging from mixtures of CERs, cholesterol, and fatty acids, to lipid precursors, alpha-hydroxy radicals, and humectants, including glycerol and urea.[9]

The most abundant AQP present in the skin is AQP3, which is located in the plasma membrane of epidermal keratinocytes which transports both water and glycerol. Aquaporin-3 transports glycerol into the SC where it acts as an endogenous humectant. Glycerol pulls water with it, creating a reservoir effect, thereby enhancing the water-holding capacity of the skin.

The expression of AQP3 channels in human skin is strongly affected by aging and long-term sun exposure, with substantially decreased levels of AQP3 in both, thereby accounting for the heightened incidence of xerosis in older individuals and/or those with skin areas that have been chronically exposed to sunlight.[4]

Consequently, the search currently is underway for compounds that can stimulate AQP3 expression, and thereby improve the hydration state of the skin by endogenous means. The herbal medicine byakkokaninjinto, an extract from the bark of *Piptadenia colubrina* (a native leguminous tree from South America), and an extract of *Ajuga turkestanica* (a plant from Central Asia) have been reported to increase AQP3 messenger RNA and/or protein levels in the skin tissue. Even urea, utilized for decades by dermatologists to treat xerosis and a key ingredient in a plethora of products, has been demonstrated to stimulate AQP3 expression in keratinocytes.

In clinical studies, the compound glyceryl glucoside,[1,10] a chemical derivative of glycerol, has been shown to promote epidermal AQP3 messenger RNA and protein upregulation, and improve skin barrier function in humans. Its inclusion in moisturizing lotions may offer an effective treatment option for dehydrated skin. The principles and indications of different classes of moisturizers are given in Table1.

Table 1: Overview of several classes of moisturizers with their indications and functions

Class	Ingredient	Function	Indications
Occlusives • Petrolatum • Dimethicone • Lanolin • Mineral oil • Jojoba oil • Olive oil	• *Petrolatum*: Most effective in treating dry skin condition • Reduces transepidermal water loss (TEWL) 99% • Penetrates deeper layer of skin to initiate lipid synthesis • *Dimethicone*: Silicone-based oil-free moisturizer, hypoallergenic but cannot reduce TEWL	Provide an occlusive, hydrophobic barrier that reduces TEWL and protects irritated inflamed skin from external irritants to promote moisture retention and allow barrier repair	Dry and/or damaged skin; formulation types include ointments and often are water-in-oil lotion or cream emulsions
Humectant Glycerin, sorbitol, urea, sodium lactate, lactic acid, carnitine, sodium pyrrolidone carboxylic acid (PCA), arginine hydrochloride, serine, alanine, histidine, citrulline, lysine, sodium chloride, glycogen, mannitol, sucrose, glutamic acid, threonine	*Glycerin*: Hygroscopic, activate transglutaminase activity in stratum corneum thereby inducing accelerated maturation of corneocytes and reduces scaling. Also modulates aquaporin-3 thereby reducing TEWL	Provide hydrating effects to the skin via humectants that attract and bind water from the deep epidermis and environment to impart hydrating benefits	Suitable for "normal" skin, maintenance of skin condition, and daily use. Can cause excessive water loss from the dermis through evaporation into the lower humidity environment. Because of this humectants are always combined with occlusives that prevent water loss Of limited help in xerotic and ichthyotic skin

Continued

Continued

Table 1: Overview of several classes of moisturizers with their indications and functions

Class	Ingredient	Function	Indications
Emollients			
Oils, lipids, and their derivatives (e.g., stearic, linoleic, linolenic, oleic, and lauric acids; cetearyl alcohol; mineral oil; lanolin)	Fatty acids in addition may influence the inflammatory cascade by producing eicosanoids	• Improve the appearance and texture of skin by filling in the crevices between corneocytes • Not designed to repair damaged skin or have long-term effects on the skin	Mostly indicated to maintain the softness of the skin. Often combined with occlusives and other therapeutic ingredients
Therapeutic			
Ceramides, PCA, glucosyl ceramide, urea, glycerin, ammonium lactate, L-lactic acid and D-lactic acid		Protect, hydrate, and support endogenous barrier repair processes	Formulated to treat xerosis and diseased skin conditions with a xerotic component; generally contain a balance of occlusives for barrier support, emollients to soften and smoothen skin, and humectants to provide water to the stratum corneum

PRINCIPLES FOR CHOOSING A MOISTURIZER TO BE USED BOTH IN XEROSIS AND ICHTHYOSIS

Since both the conditions are associated with impaired barrier function along with biochemical alteration of the SC, the ingredients in a moisturizer need to be chosen properly which will be able to supplement the defective physiomechanism. Knowledge about the interplay between ingredients in moisturizers is fundamental to get a stable and cosmetically acceptable product with preferred impact on the skin. Going beyond the traditional concept of creams, lotions and ointments with lipid and water in variable proportions, current day formularies are revolving around the incorporation of active ingredients which would actually supplement the deficit of certain molecules or actively take part in inducing physiological benefit.

Among the classes of moisturizer, the emollient-dominant and the humectant-based ones only provide temporary hydration without providing much of therapeutic benefit. Care should be taken when using these products on compromised or diseased skin, as fragrances, preservatives, and extracts can exacerbate AD in patients with symptoms of contact and inhaled allergies.

Therapeutic moisturizers are the best suited to treat xerosis and ichthyotic skin as they provide a balance of all the components to maintain the integrity of SC (Box 3). The efficacy is likely to depend on the dosage, where compliance is a great challenge faced in the management of skin diseases. Strong odor, low pH and sensory reaction may reduce patient acceptance. In addition to active substances like fats and humectants, moisturizers contain substances conventionally considered as excipients (e.g., emulsifiers, antioxidants, preservatives). Emulsifiers may weaken the barrier. Urea has been shown to reduce TEWL in atopic and ichthyotic patients. The compositon of therapeutic moisturizers are enlisted in Table 2.

Surfactants and emulsifiers modify the barrier lipids by influencing the phase behavior of the lamellae and increasing the fluidity of the lipid lamellae and facilitate the desquamatory process. Glycerol has similar effect and can be used as component of moisturizer used to treat dry skin condition. Some special things are to be considered while choosing moisturizers for ichthyotic patients (Box 4).

In dry skin conditions such as xerosis, AD, psoriasis, and others, therapeutic moisturizers that support and promote self-repair are recommended for daily use. In conditions characterized by recurrent flare-ups, moisturization is recommended to decrease the frequency of flares; as adjunctive treatment to medicinal therapy, moisturizers protect and give the skin barrier the best chance of healing. A well-constructed moisturizer should contain the key factors for hydration, which include NMF and CERs (and/or ingredients that have been

---

Box 3: Therapeutic moisturizers

- Pyrrolidone carboxylic acid
- Glyceryl glucoside
- Ceramides
- Ammonium lactate
- Alpha-hydroxy acids
- Beta-hydroxy acids
- Polyhydroxy acids
- Vitamin E, C, niacinamide
- Urea
- Panthenol

Table 2: Components of therapeutic moisturizers with function

Component	Function
Sodium pyrrolidone carboxylic acid (PCA)	• Duplicate the water-holding capacity of glycosaminoglycans in the dermis
Urea	• Disrupt hydrogen bonding, which exposes the water binding sites on the corneocytes • Promotes desquamation by dissolving the intercellular cementing substance between the corneocytes • Enhances the water-holding capacity of the stratum corneum
Alpha-hydroxy acids	• Antiaging and exfoliating property
Panthenol	• Holds and attracts water
Vitamin E	• Prevents oxidation of the polyunsaturated fatty acids of the phospholipids in the membranes by capturing singlet oxygen species • It also stabilizes the membranes against damage by phospholipase A, free fatty acids, and lysophospholipids
Ceramide	• Water modulator and a permeability barrier by forming multilayered lamellar structures with other lipids between cells in the stratum corneum layers
Glyceryl glucoside	• Promote epidermal AQP3 messenger RNA and protein upregulation and improve skin barrier function
White soft paraffin, liquid paraffin	• One of the best emollients and enhances water holding capacity of stratum corneum

---

Box 4: Special considerations while choosing the moisturizer in ichthyotic patients

- Lactic acid 5–10% and/or urea 5–10% compounded in a moisturizer base
- Combination using salicylic acid 5–10% and urea 5–10% can be compounded in either an ointment or a cream
- For keratoderma of the soles, 50% salicylic acid + 20% urea in white petroleum jelly applied nightly

---

Box 5: Side effects of moisturizers

- Contact sensitization
- Irritation
- Infection
- Systemic intoxication from propylene glycol and salicylic acid
- Acneiform eruption

---

shown to stimulate CER and barrier lipid synthesis), and modulators or enhancers of AQP expression and activity. The side effects of moisturizers are given in Box 5.

ASSESSMENT OF MOISTURIZER EFFICACY

Transepidermal water loss, one of the most common measures of efficacy, can be affected by many factors including humidity, temperature, circadian rhythms and even stress. Other limitations of TEWL estimation of moisturizer efficacy involve the devices used in its measurement.

PATIENT EDUCATION

Despite acknowledgment of the widespread benefits of emollients in the management of dry skin, they are often used incorrectly or accompanied by conflicting advice from healthcare professionals. General advice should be given on the correct and most effective method of emollient application, such as applying immediately after bathing or showering and to rub in the direction of hair growth to reduce the risk of folliculitis.

Proper advice of applying moisturizers with topical steroids should be given. Current prescribing advice recommends the corticosteroid first, followed by the emollient at least 30 minutes later.

The National Institute for Clinical Excellence (NICE) (2004) stated that emollients should not be used for 2 hours before or after the application of tacrolimus, although there are no such restrictions for pimecrolimus.

REFERENCES

1. Weber TM, Schoelermann AM, Breitenbach U, et al. Hand and foot moisturizers. In: Draelos ZD (Ed). Cosmetic Dermatology: Products and Procedures. Hoboken, NJ: Blackwell Publishing Ltd; 2010. pp. 130-8.
2. Jungersted JM, Hellgren LI, Jemec GB, et al. Lipids and skin barrier function—a clinical perspective. Contact Dermatitis. 2008;58(5):255-62.
3. Rawlings AV, Harding CR. Moisturization and skin barrier function. Dermatol Ther. 2004;17(1):43-8.
4. Grubauer G, Feingold KR, Harris RM, et al. Lipid content and lipid type as determinants of the epidermal permeability barrier. J Lipid Res. 1989;30(1):89-96.
5. Bonté F. Skin moisturization mechanisms: new data. Ann Pharm Fr. 2011;69(3):135-41.
6. Fowler J. Understanding the role of natural moisturizing factor in skin hydration. Pract Dermatol. 2012:36-40.
7. Grether-Beck S, Felsner I, Brenden H, et al. Urea uptake enhances barrier function and antimicrobial defense in humans by regulating epidermal gene expression. J Invest Dermatol. 2012;132(6):1561-72.
8. Feingold KR. Thematic review series: skin lipids. The role of epidermal lipids in cutaneous permeability barrier homeostasis. J Lipid Res. 2007;48(12):2531-46.
9. Del Rosso JQ. Factors influencing optimal skin care and product selection. In: Draelos ZD, Thaman LA (Eds). Cosmetic Formulation of Skin Care Products. New York, NY: Taylor & Francis Group; 2006. pp. 115-21.
10. Schrader A, Siefken W, Kueper T, et al. Effects of glyceryl glucoside on AQP3 expression, barrier function and hydration of human skin. Skin Pharmacol Physiol. 2012;25:192-9.

CHAPTER 9

Maintaining Skin Integrity and Moisturizers in Aged

Sidharth Sonthalia

INTRODUCTION

Dry skin or xerosis is an extremely common condition that affects people of all ages, genders and races. The basic characteristic of the disorder is the presence of rough, flaky skin that has lost its normal level of hydration and associated mechanical properties. Certain populations are at increased risk of developing dry skin and its sequel, e.g., atopic children as well as adults, people with a genetic or familial tendency of dry skin, people developing it as a result of drugs like certain cholesterol-lowering drugs, and perhaps most commonly, the elderly people. Although the degree of dry skin varies from person to person, the elderly affected with severe xerosis are prone to develop several complications including generalized and severe pruritus, eczematous conditions (typically asteatotic eczema or eczema craquelé), lichenification and secondary infection as a result of constant scratching. Dry skin *per se* impedes the patient's quality of life; and with comorbid conditions, often present in geriatric patients, aggressive moisturization is the only and the best way of preventing and treating dry skin and its complications in the elderly.

It is estimated that generalized or diffuse xerosis affects 75% of individuals over 75 years of age and is the most common cause of itching in this age group.[1] Although dry skin may affect any part of the body or may be generalized in the elderly, it is usually first noted on the lower limbs.

CLINICAL FEATURES AND COMPLICATIONS OF DRY SKIN IN THE ELDERLY

- *Dry patches of skin*: Typically over the lower limbs (Figure 1) and acral areas, soon becoming generalized (legs, hands, trunk).
- *Pruritus*: Itching is generalized, often more intense at night after a hot bath because of changes in temperature, a drop in ambient humidity, or exposure to products containing strong detergents.
- *Eczema craquelé (asteatotic eczema)*: It is characterized by intensely itchy, fissured, and cracked skin, typically over the lower limbs.
- *Secondary changes over asteatotic eczema*: Lichenification, ulceration and secondary infection due to constant scratching.

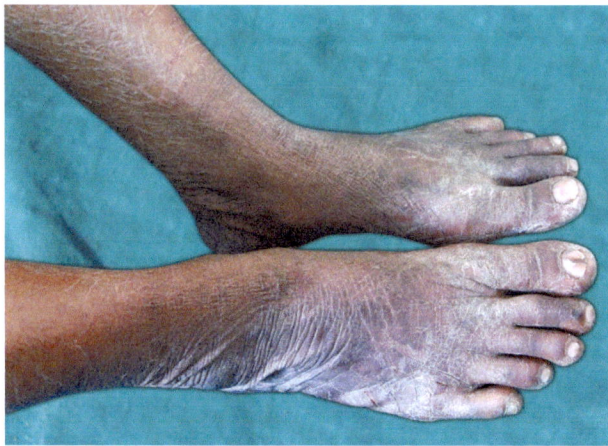

Figure 1: Severely xerotic skin over the lower limbs of a 67-year-old lady; with dry, rough, scaly skin. The changes are most pronounced over the dorsal aspect of the feet, where erythema and excoriations due to constant scratching can also be appreciated.

- *Irritant contact dermatitis*: Often due to use of cleansers/medicated soaps containing potential irritants like chloroxylenol, triclosan, *neem* derivatives, concentrated chlorhexidine, iodinated compounds, etc.

PATHOPHYSIOLOGY OF XEROSIS IN GERIATRIC POPULATION (TABLE 1)

Skin aging is associated with a number of physiologic changes that may contribute to the onset of xerosis. We may classify these factors into predisposing/facilitating factors, precipitating factors and triggering factors.

Predisposing Factors

The most common predisposing factor is a lower rate of epidermal proliferation than that of the normal skin.[2] The reduction in intercellular lipid content and natural moisturizing factor (NMF) that characterizes xerosis is both a cause and a consequence of abnormal epidermal differentiation. In fact, disruption of epidermal differentiation perpetuates the phenomenon of dry skin and further compromises the epidermal barrier. Age-related changes in collagen content give rise to a decrease in skin elasticity that heightens the sensation of dryness. A decreased senility-associated reduction in sebaceous and sweat gland activity definitely contributes further. A decline in gonadal and adrenal androgens is associated with decreased synthesis of sebum and cutaneous ceramides.[1] Last but not the least, geriatric patients who have associated atopic dermatitis (persistent or intermittent flare-ups), are at the receiving end of a higher severity of xerosis and its complications. Levels of filaggrin, the source of NMFs, are also lower in aged skin.[3]

Table 1: Pathophysiological factors implicated in xerosis in geriatric population		
Predisposing factors	**Precipitating factors**	**Triggering factors**
Senility-associated • Lower rate of epidermal proliferation • Reduction in intercellular lipid content, especially ceramides • Reduction in natural moisturizing factors • Reduction in sebaceous and sweat gland activity (hormone dependent) • Reduction in filaggrin content • Altered collagen content and structure in dermis *Other predisposing skin condition* • Atopic dermatitis (persistent or with intermittent flare-ups)	• Nutritional deficiencies • Intestinal malabsorption • Hormonal conditions: hypothyroidism, post menopausal • Chronic renal disease • Chronic liver disease • Neurologic disorders with decreased sweating • Solar radiation • Alcohol and nicotine • Medications—especially cholesterol-lowering drugs like statins • Internal malignancy • Human immunodeficiency virus infections	• Cold weather • Hot shower baths • Internal room heating without humidifiers • Ambient low humidity-based air conditioning • Overzealous use of cleansers and/or bathing without replacing natural skin emollients

Precipitating Factors

Senility is associated with a host of comorbid conditions that contribute to the overall dryness of the geriatric skin. Nutritional deficiency and intestinal malabsorption are important factors that may precipitate dryness of senile skin. Hormonal conditions, especially hypothyroidism in both genders and post-menopausal imbalance of estrogen/progesterone in women are important contributory factors. Other medical conditions such as chronic renal disease, chronic liver disease with advanced hepatic dysfunction, neurologic disorders with decreased sweating have their own mechanisms that add on to the baseline geriatric cutaneous xerosis. Agents that accelerate skin aging, such as solar radiation, alcohol and nicotine, have additional damaging effects for the skin barrier in the elderly.[3] Nicotine triggers capillary constriction, reducing blood flow and favoring the accumulation of harmful substances in the skin. Medications, especially cholesterol-lowering agents such as statins and fibrates, are often used by the elderly to keep a check on their cholesterol levels; and are well known causes of acquired xerosis and ichthyosis. Sometimes, human immunodeficiency virus (HIV) or an internal malignancy may present with severe refractory xerosis in the elderly as their first symptom.

Triggering Factors

Ambient temperature (cold weather or very hot bath), humidity (low humidity) and air conditioning of the local environment are important triggers. For example, a decrease in ambient humidity has been shown to reduce the generation of free amino acids in the stratum corneum (SC) and increase skin dryness.[4] Overzealous use of cleansers and/or bathing without replacing natural skin emollients is fairly common in the elderly; often due to lack of proper dermatological guidance.

MANAGEMENT OF DRY SKIN AND COMPLICATIONS IN GERIATRIC POPULATION

General Care

There are a number of general measures that reduce the propensity of dry skin in the elderly. Advise patients to drink sufficient water (but preventing fluid overload in patients with cardiac dysfunction), and a balanced diet (with predominance of hydrated fruits and vegetables such as melons) to ensure the essential nutritional intake required to maintain epidermal homeostasis. Physical exercise (appropriate for the age) stimulates blood circulation, thereby increasing the transfer of nutrients and oxygen to the keratinocytes.[1] It also favors epithelial regeneration, strengthens connective tissue, and increases collagen production. Advice about cessation of smoking and alcohol, and minimizing exposure to sunlight should be given. Instead of irritating soaps, they should use soaps or shower gels (with an acidic pH and containing humectants) without overzealous use of a loofah or any rubbing or sponging. Addition of a pinch of baking soda in their bathing water may also be helpful. Availability of bath oils has made bathing protocols for the elderly more convenient and effective prevention against xerosis.

Specific Skin Care Regimens

- The *three-step moisturizing protocol* (author's personal terminology) has been found to be very useful for the elderly with dry skin
    - *Step 1*: Gentle bathing with a non-irritating, humectant-based and pH-balanced soap or shower gel, with or without use of bath oils mixed in the bathing water
    - *Step 2*: After bathing, aqua-based lotion or cream that have both hydrating and humectant properties (containing NMFs, such as urea) should be applied directly over moist skin within 2–3 minutes; without toweling. Toweling the skin dry is known to increase intercellular lipid loss
    - *Step 3*: Application of a lipid-based emollient over-and-above the aqua-based lotion not only prevents transepidermal water loss (TEWL), by forming a practically impermeable sealing layer (as an occlusive); but additionally provides raw material (in the form of lipids) for the Odland bodies to regenerate intrinsic stratum corneal lipid balance. Such lipid-based emollients should ideally contain a mixture of lipids like ceramides, free sterols, essential and non-essential free fatty acids, and cholesterol. Ceramides are the principal source of essential fatty acids, of which, linoleic acid is the most important
- Avoidance of fragranced colognes, creams, and lotions (especially if they are alcohol-based) owing to their SC dehydrating properties
- Fabric: Patients should wear soft fabrics, preferably natural and pure cotton to minimize friction that could exacerbate xerosis. Detergents or fabric softeners used in laundry should be specifically designed to be gentle on the skin.[3] Tight clothing should be avoided since increased friction may exacerbate xerosis.

Topical Treatment

Topical application of the components to re-establish normal keratinocyte differentiation should contain active ingredients that rapidly penetrate the epidermis to stimulate the production pathways of intercellular lipids. This "inside out" approach, compared to the traditional "outside in" approach, appears to produce more effective therapeutic outcomes.[3] The topical preparations designed to treat dry skin are emollients or hydrating substances, humectants, and occlusives; available in preparations such as lotions or creams or ointments. Creams may further be oil-in-water (O/W) emulsions (higher concentration of oil than water) or water-in-oil (W/O) emulsions (higher concentration of water than oil).

Repair of the Lipid Barrier

The need for the supply of three essential physiological lipids (ceramides, cholesterol, free fatty acids) through commercial emollients needs no over-emphasis. These physiologic lipids have several advantages over nonphysiologic molecules; since they penetrate SC more easily, and function as structural elements in the epidermal barrier and trigger epidermal repair.

Supply and Retention of Water in the SC

A "humectant" is a substance (often complex mixture of active ingredients or special combinations of amino acids, hydrocarbon, silicones) that attracts and retains water; playing a passive role from the outside. A "hydrant" (e.g., glycerin or propylene glycol), on the other hand, is one that actively supplies and restores water to the skin by their hygroscopic property. Humectants like *glycerol* are capable of correcting defects in skin elasticity and barrier function (independent of lipid loss). One of those mechanisms is by inducing reduction of synthesis of aquaporin-3, an epidermal water/glycerol transporter that tends to dehydrate SC.[3,5] It is, therefore, recommended that topical moisturizers should include this substance.

Alleviation of Pruritus

Since, pruritus and complications of scratching due to xerosis are appalling for the elderly, topical application of antipruritic agents, apart from moisturization is often helpful, especially during bouts of intense itching that elderly encounter during the temperature/humidity changes or at night. Products containing glycine (that blocks the release of histamine from the mast cells), calamine and aloe vera (that soothen the skin), and mild counterirritant containing moisturizers (e.g., with 0.5% menthol and 0.5% camphor), aid in breaking the self-perpetuating itch-scratch cycle. By blocking the mast cell release of histamine, glycine interferes with the release of the mediators of the inflammation-itch phenomenon.[6] Topical corticosteroid preparations have an indirect effect on itching as they improve the condition of the skin; but are better used to treat a complication such as an evolving or established xerotic eczema, rather than as a general "antipruritic", since extensive and prolonged use of topical corticosteroids can cause a plethora of undesirable side effects, especially skin atrophy (Figure 2) and increased skin fragility.

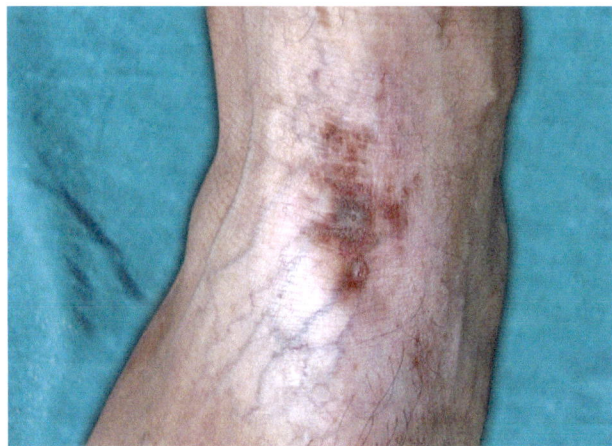

Figure 2: Steroid-modified lichen simplex chronicus over the dorsum of the ankle (in a background of xerosis) of a 65-year-old patient, with evidence of prolonged topical steroid abuse—skin atrophy, dyschromia and telangiectasias.

Repair of the Stratum Corneum

Substances like dexpanthenol stimulate and accelerate the process of epidermal regeneration. Dexpanthenol promotes fibroblast proliferation as well as migration and stimulates intracellular protein synthesis.[3] Addition of low concentration alpha-hydroxy acids has also been found to facilitate desquamation and improve lipid biosynthesis.[7] However, in view of their topically irritating action, they should be combined with other emollients such as cetylated fatty esters, to make them soothing.

Multipronged Approach to Managing Geriatric Xerosis: The "Ideal" Moisturizer

Topical preparations for the treatment of dry skin, especially in the elderly should contain molecules that provide effective water supply and retention in SC, restore the lipid content of SC by providing them from outside as well as stimulating intrinsic synthesis by Odland bodies, activate the epidermal barrier repair mechanisms if the barrier has been breached and stimulate intrinsic epidermal regeneration process. Table 2 enumerates the active ingredients that should be included in any formulation for an "ideal" topical moisturizing preparation for ensuring the perfect moisturization for geriatric population. The so-called ideal formulation would contain hydrants (such as amino acids), physiologic humectant (glycerol), physiologic lipids (ceramides, cholesterol, free fatty acids), antipruritic agent (glycerol or glycine), and a component that enhances epidermal differentiation (like dexpanthenol).[3]

Other ingredients that have been suggested to play additional role in correction of xerosis include: oats (rich in water, proteins, lipids, mineral salts, and vitamins; with hydrating, antipruritic, and anti-inflammatory activities), allantoin (hydrating, keratoplastic and conditioning properties), α-bisabolol

Table 2: Components and functions of the "ideal" moisturizer

Active component	Examples	Function
Hydrating agents	• Polyols: Glycerol, sorbitol, propylene glycol • NMF: Urea • Reconstituted NMFs: Mixture of amino acids, sodium lactate, lactate acid, citrate • Hyaluronic acid	• Hydrate the stratum corneum by supplying water molecules • Some molecules promote corneodesmolysis to maintain epidermal desquamation • Restore and maintain skin elasticity and flexibility
Humectants	• Hydrocarbons (paraffin and Vaseline) • Fatty oils and alcohols (glycerol, propylene glycol) • Colloid substances [cellulose derivatives, polymers, e.g., xanthan gum (natural), carbopol (synthetic)] • Silicones	• Attract water molecules from the environment and deeper layer of the skin and passively retain them in stratum corneum
Physiologic lipids	• Ceramides • Cholesterol • Free fatty acids especially linoleic acid	• Replace the lost stratum corneum lipids • Provide material for intrinsic stratum corneum synthesis of natural lipids to reinforce epidermal differentiation and barrier function by restoring corneocyte cohesion
Antipruritic agents	• Glycine • Glycerol • Calamine	• To alleviate xerosis-related itching and break the itch-scratch cycle
Epidermal "enhancers"	• Dexpanthenol • Alpha-hydroxy acids	• Promote fibroblast proliferation, migration and stimulates intracellular protein synthesis; resulting in enhanced epidermal differentiation
Excipient	• Water-rich: Facial skin, acute eczemas, summer season • Lipid-rich: Trunk, limbs and body folds, chronic lichenified eczemas, winter season	

NMF, natural moisturizing factor.

(emollient, antimicrobial and anti-inflammatory activities), aloe vera (soothing and emollient), and glycyrrhetic acid (anti-inflammatory and emollient). Apart from these, many new compounds are under preparation and testing, before they find their way into the commercial market of moisturizers, especially catering to geriatric xerosis.

CONCLUSION

Dry skin and its complications can indeed be very frustrating for the geriatric population with significant impact on their quality of life. Abnormal epidermal differentiation being the main predisposing factor for geriatric xerosis, is frequently accompanied with comorbid medical conditions and other precipitating and triggering factors that worsen the dryness. Proper counseling about general care to prevent loss of skin's water and lipid contents, with judicious selection and generous use of a good moisturizer, are instrumental in both preventing and treating dry skin in the elderly.

REFERENCES

1. Barco D, Giménez-Arnau A. Xerosis: a dysfunction of the epidermal barrier. Actas Dermosifiliogr. 2008;99(9):671-82.
2. Engelke M, Jensen JM, Ekanayake-Mudiyanselage S, et al. Effects of xerosis and ageing on epidermal proliferation and differentiation. Br J Dermatol. 1997;137(2):219-25.
3. Proksch E, Lachapelle JM. The management of dry skin with topical emollients--recent perspectives. J Dtsch Dermatol Ges. 2005;3(10):768-74.
4. Katagiri C, Sato J, Nomura J, et al. Changes in environmental humidity affect the water-holding property of the stratum corneum and its free amino acid content, and the expression of the filaggrin in the epidermis of hairless mice. J Dermatol Sci. 2003;31(1):29-35.
5. Hara M, Verkman AS. Glycerol replacement corrects defective skin hydration, elasticity and barrier function in aquaporin-3-deficient mice. Proc Natl Acad Sci U S A. 2003;100(12):7360-5.
6. Paubert-Braquet M, Lefrançois G, Picquot S. Etude in vitro du pouvoir antiprurigineux du glycocolle: effet sur la dégranulation des mastocytes. Thérapeutique. 1992;95:2-3.
7. Rawlings AV, Matts PJ. Stratum corneum moisturization at the molecular level: an update in relation to the dry skin cycle. J Invest Dermatol. 2005;124(6):1099-110.

CHAPTER 10

Steroid-Sparing Emollients in Dermatology

Koushik Lahiri, Abhijit Saha, Shilpa Garg

INTRODUCTION

Topical corticosteroids (TCS) and emollients are cornerstones of management of different inflammatory and eczematous dermatoses. Intermittent use of TCS is particularly effective in controlling acute flares and discontinuation may lead to exacerbation of the condition. Topical corticosteroids due to their rapid absorption and anti-inflammatory action can calm an inflamed skin and are especially used for the swift resolution of acute flares in psoriasis, atopic dermatitis (AD) and eczema. Different preparations with varied potencies and vehicles are available in market and their choice depends upon the age of the patient and site and severity of involvement. With due consideration to the beneficial role of TCS, cutaneous side effects such as atrophy, telangiectasia, striae, hypopigmentation, hyperpigmentation, steroid rosacea, steroid acne, steroid-induced folliculitis, tinea incognito, perioral dermatitis, tachyphylaxis and hirsutism due to long-term continuous unsupervised use of these molecules cannot be disregarded. Even systemic absorption, though very minimal, under certain circumstances may lead to growth retardation in children, cataract and glaucoma in adults and obviously hypothalamic-pituitary-adrenal axis suppression.

With this background, the need of an alternative pharmacological agent with barrier repair and anti-inflammatory property is obvious. Emollients, whether over-the-counter (OTC) colloidal oat meal or petrolatum or newly introduced medical device cream, probably are the best fit in this regard and can be used indefinitely without aforementioned associated risks.

Grimalt et al. compared the efficacy of an emollient containing oat extract with the amount of steroid required to treat moderate-to-severe AD.[1] Compared to the control group (without emollient) requirement of moderate-to-high potent steroid was reduced significantly in emollient group in 6-week study period. Another study showed that application of TCS every other day along with the test cream is equally effective as once or twice daily application of steroid alone.[2] Emollients can also reduce relapse after cessation of TCS therapy.[3,4] A country wide multicentric study on topical steroid abuse has comprehensively enlisted all the aspects of this menace.[5] A study found that daily morning application of hydrocortisone 2.5% cream combined with once daily evening application of water-in-oil emollient cream was equally efficacious as twice daily application of hydrocortisone 2.5% cream in children with AD.[6] Similarly, an open labeled study of 96 patients with chronic plaque psoriasis found that once daily application of betamethasone dipropionate cream along with a water-in-oil based moisturizing cream or lotion was equally efficacious as twice daily application of betamethasone dipropionate cream.[7] Also once daily application of both betamethasone dipropionate cream together with a water-in-oil based cream or lotion was significantly better than once daily application of betamethasone dipropionate cream alone ($p = 0.05$). The study concluded that water-in-oil emollients were useful in the treatment of chronic plaque psoriasis and provided a steroid-sparing effect. A study demonstrated that addition of an emollient containing water, petrolatum, shea butter, evening primrose oil, glycerin, paraffin oil, niacinamide, butylene glycol, benzoic acid, carbomer and also specific active Rhealba® oat extracts (flavonoids and saponins) significantly reduced the use of desonide 0.1% cream in infants with AD.[8] Hence, moisturizers can provide an alternative to corticosteroids as an intermittent therapy in order to limit the localized side effects of corticosteroids and can be of great help as a steroid-sparing agent.

EPIDERMAL BARRIER DYSFUNCTION

Certain inflammatory dermatoses are associated with a defective skin barrier function and stratum corneum hydration. Disruption of epidermal barrier can lead to increased density of epidermal Langerhans cells, enhance the inflammatory responses by increasing the presentation of foreign antigen and decreased antimicrobial peptides which play an important role in the innate skin defense.

Epidermal barrier dysfunction classically described in AD is multifactorial. In a state of physiological balance, corneocytes are surrounded by continuous phase of ceramide (50%), cholesterol (25%) and free fatty acids (10–20%) in certain proportion leading to formation of so-called "brick and mortar" model. In AD, there is a reduced formation and organization of all the lipid components, especially ceramide leading to formation of a defective lipid mortar. In this regard, role of filaggrin, a structural protein essential for corneocyte adhesion and formation of cornified envelope should be considered. Filaggrin also acts as a source of natural moisturizing factor essential for corneocyte hydration. This may explain increased transepidermal water loss (TEWL) in AD patients with filaggrin mutation than those without such mutation. Other contributing factors are alteration of antimicrobial barrier, increased production of serine proteases and mast cell chymase.

The ultimate outcomes of this defective epidermal barrier are increased TEWL resulting in dry skin, predisposition to secondary infection, sustained ingress of antigens, increased density of epidermal Langerhans cells and release of proinflammatory cytokines (Th2 dominant) which are prerequisite for initiation as well as perpetuation of inflammation. This "outside-to-inside" view of AD pathogenesis reasonably established skin barrier dysfunction as a primary event, which was previously thought to be secondary event downstream to the consequences of primary immunological alterations; inside-to-outside view of AD pathogenesis.

Understanding the role of epidermal barrier has brought about the concept that along with treatment of inflammation, restoration of skin barrier is equally important which further prevent penetration of allergens and irritants, thus putting a brake on the vicious cycle. Emollients are ideal candidates in this regard with their steroid-sparing effect when used regularly and liberally.

MOISTURIZER AS STEROID-SPARING AGENT

Petrolatum was initially thought to be a solely occlusive agent by virtue of formation of epidermal impermeable barrier, thus preventing TEWL. Further studies found that petrolatum permeate through the stratum corneum interstices and accelerate barrier recovery. It imparts a soft and silky feel to the skin. However, they are not very cosmetically appealing to the patients due to their greasy feel. Miller DW et al. compared efficacy and cost effectiveness of a glycyrrhetinic acid containing barrier repair cream, a ceramide-dominant barrier repair cream and an OTC-petrolatum based moisturizer as monotherapy in mild-to-moderate AD in children.[9] The result showed no statistically significant difference in efficacy among these three products; rather OTC-petrolatum was found to be 47 times cost effective than rest. Another study reflected the same; parity between a prescription device [containing lamellar matrix that mimic the normal skin barrier (triglycerides, phospholipids, and squalene) along with the anti-inflammatory cannabinoid N-palmitoylethanolamine (N-PEA), an endogenous fatty acid amide which inhibits mast cell activation] and mineral oil, paraffin and petrolatum-based traditional moisturizer in the treatment of mild-to-moderate symmetrical eczema of hand and leg.[10] A study demonstrated comparable efficacy of a barrier repair cream containing petrolatum as a primary ingredient to topical calcineurin inhibitor.[11]

Dimethicone is an occlusive agent which is a mixture of polydimethylsiloxanes and silicon dioxide. It is a safe and effective skin moisturizing ingredient, though it is not as effective as petrolatum in reducing TEWL. It helps in reducing irritation associated with inflammatory diseases such as AD and allergic contact dermatitis. Barrier creams containing combination of cyclomethicone (a cyclic higher-viscosity silicone) and dimethicone help to prevent sensitization of skin to allergens, and hence is useful in decreasing symptoms of itching and burning associated with contact dermatitis. A study demonstrated significant reduction in the incidence of incontinence associated dermatitis seen in patients using dimethicone-impregnated clothes.[12]

Colloidal oatmeal is the colloidal extract of finely grinded particle of oat and contains various active components like polysaccharides, proteins, lipids, saponins, enzymes, flavonoids, vitamins and avenanthramides (polyphenol). It has been approved by US Food and Drug Administration (FDA) in the monograph of skin protectant drug in 2003. It is helpful in the treatment of dermatologic conditions which are associated with symptoms of itch and irritation due to their ability to soothe and protect the inflamed skin. Ready-to-use oatmeal preparations contain concentrated starch-protein fraction of the oat grain mixed with emollient. Fine particles of oatmeal disperse on the skin to form a protective occlusive barrier which prevents water loss and moisturizes the skin leading to improvement in skin barrier. Oatmeal saponins may help to normalize the skin pH by solubilizing dirt, oil and sebaceous secretions. Oats also possess antioxidant, ultraviolet absorbent and anti-inflammatory properties which are due to its ferulic acid, caffeic acid, coumaric acid, flavonoids and α-tocopherol components. It also contains avenanthramides (phenolic compounds) which has anti-inflammatory, hydrating and antipruritic action by decreasing the production of nuclear factor-kappa B in keratinocytes, reducing the proinflammatory cytokine production such as interleukin (IL)-8 and inhibiting prostaglandin synthesis.

Ceramides are an essential component of the normal stratum corneum and functions to maintain the skin barrier. Changes in ceramide are seen in patients with AD. Application of moisturizers is known to reduce the frequency of flares in AD and also helps to limit the need for TCS, probably due to recovery of barrier. A study demonstrated equivalent improvement in the signs and symptoms of AD with an emollient containing ceramide and hyaluronic acid as compared to pimecrolimus.[13] Another study showed significant improvement in the symptoms of AD with a ceramide dominant barrier repair emollient as compared to an OTC moisturizer in a study of 24 children with recalcitrant AD who were also receiving either TCS or topical calcineurin inhibitor.[14] So it is difficult to say confidently that better looking severity scoring of AD (SCORAD) is solely due to replacement of OTC moisturizer with ceramide dominant barrier repair emollient. A study reported similar efficacy between a preparation containing combination of ceramides, cholesterol and fatty acids (in the ratio of 3:1:1 and containing capric acid, cholesterol, conjugated linolenic acid, candelilla and petrolatum) and mid-potency TCS.[15,16] In a multicenter, investigator-blinded, randomized trial, a preparation containing ceramide, capric acid, conjugated linolenic acid and cholesterol as main ingredients was compared to fluticasone cream in 121 patients with moderate-to-severe AD and showed reduction in clinical disease severity and pruritus and improvement in sleep habits at both 14 and 28 days after initiation of treatment. Although patients on fluticasone improved faster and had greater improvement by day 14, both the groups showed equal efficacy by day 28.[17] Again the missing link is lack of an age matched control group treated solely on traditional moisturizer. In another study, preparation containing ceramide, capric acid, conjugated linolenic acid and cholesterol as main ingredients was tested as monotherapy or in combination with additional therapy in mild-to-moderate AD. Interestingly, subjects were directly involved in the study and 71% of them denied requirement of any additional treatment. Again, this study lacks any moisturizer comparator.[18] A more recent study established efficacy of a new moisturizer containing filaggrin breakdown product.[19]

Topical corticosteroids induced atrophic changes in skin, such as thinning of the epidermis and decrease in dermal ground substance, can be minimized by application of 12% ammonium lactate. Ammonium lactate is a humectant which increases the thickness of epidermis and amount of dermal glycosaminoglycans. A study evaluated the effects of clobetasol propionate, 12% ammonium lactate, and both agents together on skin atrophy and found that 12% ammonium lactate produced significant sparing of both epidermal and dermal atrophy without influencing the bioavailability or anti-inflammatory properties of clobetasol propionate.[20]

Additional ingredients such as glycerin, urea, hydroxy acids and propylene glycol are other common humectants which are added to OTC ingredients in order to increase the ability of the skin to absorb water. Glycerol/glycerin is most effective and has the ability to activate enzyme transglutaminase in the stratum corneum, leading to accelerated maturation of corneocytes as well as increasing aquaporins (particularly aquaporin-3) in diseased skin, which results in increases, in skin hydration and reduction in TEWL. A double-blinded study showed efficacy and tolerability of 5% urea moisturizer and 10% urea lotion in the treatment of AD.[21] Another study demonstrated use of 5% urea to prolong disease-free interval in cases of controlled hand eczema.[22] Loden M concluded that urea containing moisturizers help in barrier repair most probably by decreasing TEWL.[23]

Prescription moisturizers are not considered as drug, rather medical devices approved by FDA. The approval process is less cumbersome and expensive than regular drug approval and more focused on safety than efficacy. It is more appropriate to designate them as 510(k) cleared where clearance is based on capability to reduce TEWL. In addition to their barrier repair property, they possess anti-inflammatory and antipruritic properties which contribute to their steroid-sparing effect in the treatment of inflammatory dermatoses.

Top in the list is Atopiclair® which contains *Butyrospermum parkii* (shea butter), glycyrrhetinic acid 2%, *Vitis vinifera* (grapevine) extract, hyaluronic acid, bisabolol (German chamomile) and telmesteine. Few multicentric, randomized, vehicle-controlled studies were carried out which demonstrated safety and efficacy of Atopiclair® as a monotherapy in the treatment of mild-to-moderate AD in both pediatric and adult population. All the studies showed that the test cream is significantly more effective than vehicle alone. Again there is lack of data comparing Atopiclair® with OTC moisturizers.

Second in the list is MimyX™ which contains lamellar matrix that mimics the normal skin barrier (triglycerides, phospholipids, and squalene) along with the anti-inflammatory cannabinoid N-PEA, an endogenous fatty acid amide which inhibits mast cell activation.

Third in the list is Eletone® emulsion which has a high lipid content dispersed in an outer aqueous phase (Hydrolipid Technology™) in petrolatum, purified water, and mineral oil. In an investigator-blinded bilateral study, authors claimed that Eletone® is equally effective as 1% pimecrolimus cream in the treatment of AD.[11]

Hylatopic Plus®, fourth in the list contains hyaluronic acid, *Theobroma grandiflorum* seed butter, glycerin, petrolatum, and tocopheryl acetate (vitamin E) and dimethicone.

Medical device creams containing emollients and agents with anti-inflammatory and antipruritic properties are used for the treatment of inflammatory dermatoses and help in treating the epidermal barrier dysfunction and in limiting the potential of long-term use of TCS. Agents like *B. parkii* (shea tree), glycyrrhetinic acid (licorice), *V. vinifera* (grapevine) extract, bisabolol (German chamomile), hyaluronic acid and tocopheryl acetate (vitamin E) are added and are thought to have moisturizing, anti-inflammatory and antioxidant properties. These agents can help in relieving the burning, itching and pain experienced with various dermatoses including AD, allergic contact dermatitis and radiation dermatitis and also provide relief from dry skin. Ingredient like telmesteine prevents epidermal breakdown by inhibiting elastase, collagenase and matrix metalloproteinases. Lipid components like triglycerides, phospholipids, and squalene are helpful as they mimic the normal skin barrier. N-palmitoylethanolamine is an anti-inflammatory cannabinoid. It is an endogenous fatty acid amide which is thought to target the peroxisome proliferator-activated receptor-alpha. Ingredients such as purified water, olive oil, glycerin, pentylene glycol, vegetable oil, and hydrogenated lecithin provide humectant and emollient effects. Other ingredients which are utilized in such preparations are ceramide, conjugated linoleic acid, mineral oil, cholesterol, palmitic acid, *Euphorbia cerifera* (candelilla) wax, *T. grandiflorum* seed butter, corn syrup solids, squalene, glycerin, petrolatum, and dimethicone.

An adequate quantity of emollient should be prescribed for optimal effect (250–500 g/week in patients with AD).[24,25] Studies state that for maximum steroid-sparing benefit, emollients should be applied in a ratio of 10:1 with steroid.[24,25] Few authors recommend weekender approach where patient applies TCS only on weekends and emollients during the weekdays. Emollients can act as a steroid-sparing agent in various dermatological disorders provided the patient is educated well regarding its use.

CONCLUSION

From the above discussion, it is evident that OTC-emollients or prescription moisturizers are important therapeutic options for treatment of inflammatory dermatoses. Their anti-inflammatory and antipruritic property definitely play role for their steroid-sparing effect. Their barrier repair property further acts synergistically to halt the pathological processes. Darker side of the story need to be enlightened, is the paucity of evidence-based support in favor of superiority of medical device creams over traditional OTC moisturizers. But at this moment, at least it can be said with certainty that both of them are effective to restore skin barrier.

Lastly, it is the judicious use of TCS and liberal use of emollient which can provide proper "healing touch" to the patients suffering from various inflammatory dermatoses. Only proper harmony between lyrics and tunes makes a song perfect. And at the end of the day, nothing can be more satisfactory to a treating physician than bringing a smile to the patient.

REFERENCES

1. Grimalt R, Mengeaud V, Cambazard F. The steroid-sparing effect of an emollient therapy in infants with atopic dermatitis: a randomized controlled study. Dermatology. 2007;214(1):61-7.
2. Msika P, De Belilovsky C, Piccardi N, et al. New emollient with topical corticosteroid-sparing effect in treatment of childhood atopic dermatitis: SCORAD and quality of life improvement. Pediatr Dermatol. 2008;25:606-12.
3. Seite S, Khemis A, Rougier A, et al. Emollient for maintenance therapy after topical corticotherapy in mild psoriasis. Exp Dermatol. 2009;18(12):1076-8.
4. Cassano N, Mantegazza R, Battaglini S, et al. Adjuvant role of a new emollient cream in patients with palmar and/or plantar psoriasis: a pilot randomized open-label study. G Ital Dermatol Venereol. 2010;145(6):789-92.

5. Saraswat A. Topical corticosteroid use in children: Adverse effects and how to minimize them. Indian J Dermatol Venereol Leprol. 2010;76(3):225-8.
6. Lucky AW, Leach AD, Laskarzewski P, et al. Use of an emollient as a steroid sparing agent in the treatment of mild to moderate atopic dermatitis in children. Pediatr Dermatol. 1997;14(4):321-4.
7. Watsky KL, Freije L, Leneveu MC, et al. Water-in-oil emollients as steroid sparing adjunctive therapy in the treatment of psoriasis. Cutis. 1992;50(5):383-6.
8. Grimalt R, Mengeaud V, Cambazard F, et al. The steroid-sparing effect of an emollient therapy in infants with atopic dermatitis: a randomized controlled study. Dermatology. 2007;214(1):61-7.
9. Miller DW, Koch SB, Yentzer BA, et al. An over-the-counter moisturizer is as clinically effective as, and more cost-effective than, prescription barrier creams in the treatment of children with mild-to-moderate atopic dermatitis: a randomized, controlled trial. J Drugs Dermatol. 2011;10(5):531-7.
10. Draelos ZD. An evaluation of prescription device moisturizers. J Cosmet Dermatol. 2009;8(1):40-3.
11. Emer JJ, Frankel A, Sohn A, et al. A bilateral comparison study of pimecrolimus cream 1% and a topical medical device cream in the treatment of patients with atopic dermatitis. J Drugs Dermatol. 2011;10(7):735-43.
12. Beeckman D, Verhaeghe S, Defloor T, et al. A 3-in-1 perineal care washcloth impregnated with dimethicone 3% versus water and pH neutral soap to prevent and treat incontinence-associated dermatitis: a randomized, controlled clinical trial. J Wound Ostomy Continence Nurs. 2011;38(6):627-34.
13. Frankel A, Sohn A, Patel RV, et al. Bilateral comparison study of pimecrolimus cream 1% and a ceramide-hyaluronic acid emollient foam in the treatment of patients with atopic dermatitis. J Drugs Dermatol. 2011;10(6):666-72.
14. Chamlin SL, Kao J, Frieden IJ, et al. Ceramide-dominant barrier repair lipids alleviate childhood atopic dermatitis: changes in barrier function provide a sensitive indicator of disease activity. J Am Acad Dermatol. 2002;47(2):198-208.
15. Madaan A. Epiceram for the treatment of atopic dermatitis. Drugs Today (Barc). 2008;44(10):751-5.
16. Bikowski J. Case studies assessing a new skin barrier repair cream for the treatment of atopic dermatitis. J Drugs Dermatol. 2009;8(11):1037-41.
17. Sugarman JL, Parish LC. Efficacy of a lipid-based barrier repair formulation in moderate-to-severe pediatric atopic dermatitis. J Drugs Dermatol. 2009;8(12):1106-11.
18. Kircik LH, Del Rosso JQ, Aversa D. Evaluating clinical use of a ceramide-dominant, physiologic lipid-based topical emulsion for atopic dermatitis. J Clin Aesthet Dermatol. 2011;4:34-40.
19. Simpson E, Böhling A, Bielfeldt S, et al. Improvement of skin barrier function in atopic dermatitis patients with a new moisturizer containing a ceramide precursor. J Dermatolog Treat. 2013;24(2):122-5.
20. Lavker RM, Kaidbey K, Leyden JJ. Effects of topical ammonium lactate on cutaneous atrophy from a potent topical corticosteroid. J Am Acad Dermatol. 1992;26(4):535-44.
21. Bissonnette R, Maari C, Provost N, et al. A double-blind study of tolerance and efficacy of a new urea-containing moisturizer in patients with atopic dermatitis. J Cosmet Dermatol. 2010;9(1):16-21.
22. Wiren K, Nohlgard C, Nyberg F, et al. Treatment with a barrier-strengthening moisturizing cream delays relapse of atopic dermatitis: a prospective and randomized controlled clinical trial. J Eur Acad Dermatol Venereol. 2009;23(11):1267-72.
23. Loden M. Urea-containing moisturizers influence barrier properties of normal skin. Arch Dermatol Res. 1996;288(2):103-7.
24. Primary Care Dermatology Society and British Association of Dermatologists. Guidelines on the Management of Atopic Eczema, Vol. 39. Berkhamsted: Medendium Group Publishing; 2009. pp. 399-402.
25. Cork MJ, Britton J, Butler L, et al. Comparison of parent knowledge, therapy utilization and severity of atopic eczema before and after explanation and demonstration of topical therapies by a specialist dermatology nurse. Br J Dermatol. 2003;149(3):582-9.

CHAPTER 11

Neonatal and Infantile Skin Care and Moisturizers

Indrashis Podder, Rashmi Sarkar

INTRODUCTION

The skin of a neonate or infant differs conspicuously from the adult skin (Table 1). It is more susceptible to trauma and infections, thus requiring special care. Given the delicate nature of neonatal and infantile skin, most experts opine to avoid the use of any substance on their skin without careful consideration of their potential hazards,[1] however use of certain substances, like moisturizers, become a necessity for proper baby skin care in harsh climatic conditions. This chapter focuses on some of the important ingredients of proper skin care and also their utilities in this age group.

PRINCIPLES OF SKIN CARE OF THE NEONATES AND INFANTS

Some important principles which guide the proper neonatal and infantile skin care deserve special mention:
- *Prevention of infections*: The neonatal and infantile skin has increased susceptibility of infection, especially from coagulase-negative *Staphylococci* (CONS) and *Staphylococcus aureus*,[2] mainly affecting the axilla, groin, other body folds and scalp. Thus, proper and judicious use of cleansers

Table 1: Differences between neonatal/infantile skin and adult skin		
Features	**Neonatal/infantile skin**	**Adult skin**
Structure	• Thinner epidermis • Less cohesion between epidermis and dermis • Dermis is thinner with less elastic fibers	• Normal epidermis • Good cohesion between epidermis and dermis • Fully developed elastic fibers
Sweat glands	Decreased sweating capacity	Full sweating
Hair	Lanugo/vellus hair	Vellus and terminal hair
Permeability	Increased permeability to fat soluble substances and increased absorption due to higher surface area to body weight ratio	Good resistance to penetration

and moisturizers along with adequate hydration and avoidance of friction becomes a necessity to avoid the menace of infections.
- *Bathing the newborn*: Bathing with lukewarm water (temperature < 37°C) is an essential way of cleansing the newborn skin, however it should only be given once the body temperature has stabilized and the neonate is hemodynamically stable. Usually, the first bath is given 2–6 hours after birth in a healthy term baby (> 2,500 g),[3] however delayed bathing is necessary in certain situations viz. low-birth-weight infant, winter season, etc.[1]

IMPORTANT SKIN CARE AGENTS—AT A GLANCE

Some important substances which can be used for proper skin care in this population are given below. However, all agents should be used with extreme caution given the delicate nature of their skin, and physician consultation is a must to avoid any complication.
- *Emollients/moisturizers/lubricants*: These are agents which soften and smoothen the skin (plasticizer of the epidermis) by restoring water to the skin for a short period or help it retain moisture when applied after bathing. Humectants like lactic acid and urea may be added to the emollients to enhance their efficacy. Although some emollients can cause contact dermatitis[4] (e.g., mustard oil), recent studies show use of emollients from birth may play a role to prevent the development of atopic dermatitis as they may improve barrier function if used judiciously.[5] These moisturizers/emollients can be of the following types:[6]
  - *Hydrocarbons*: Most effective, although least cosmetically acceptable; e.g., vaseline, paraffin, petrolatum, mineral and "baby" oils, etc. Petrolatum is commonly used in several baby emollients and seems to work well
  - *Oil-in-water (O/W) emulsions (creams)*: Second most effective. Contain oils, fatty alcohols, waxes with emulsifiers and humectants; e.g., cold creams, skin oil (Nivea), etc.
  - *Water-in-oil (W/O) emulsions (ointments)*: Least effective but most comfortable to use. Principally contain water along with emulsifiers, colors, fragrances, preservatives and humectants
  - *Oils*: In the Indian scenario, vegetable oils are extensively used for massage and as moisturizers.

Coconut oil is preferred to mustard oil (it may cause contact dermatitis due to presence of allylisothiocyanate antigen), e.g., mineral oil, vegetable oils viz. coconut oil, palm kernel oil, mustard oil, olive oil, synthetic oil.

Note: Although a variety of compounds like aloe, jojoba oil and vitamin E have been used as folk remedies for many years and have garnered commercial attention as lubricants, their precise role is yet to be elucidated.

- *Role of sunflower oil and olive oil in newborn period*: Although, a wide variety of natural oils have been used in the neonatal period to nourish the skin, recent studies have shown all natural oils are not beneficial. While sunflower oil has been shown to enhance the integrity of stratum corneum and hydration of skin, olive oil has shown detrimental effects on the neonatal skin (impairing skin barrier, enhancing chance of atopic dermatitis; production of erythema).[7] Sunflower oil massage has also led to reduced mortality among

preterm neonates in developing countries.[8] Thus, contrary to the popular belief that all natural oils are beneficial for the skin, we now know sunflower oil is better than olive oil. The use of latter should be discouraged.
- *Cleansing agents*: Cleansers are substances which help to remove dirt, bacteria, dead skin cells and other debri from the skin surface. Ideally, a baby cleanser should be devoid of fragrance to avoid irritation. However, Lavender et al.[9] found no superiority of cleansers when compared to water in this regard. Broadly cleansers are of four types:[1]
  - Alkaline soaps (make skin dry, rough, flaky, tight)
  - Acidic or neutral synthetic detergents (syndets) (less irritating and milder than soaps; do not alter skin pH)
  - Special soaps, e.g., superfatted soaps
  - The fourth type is emollient cleansers which contain bath additives with mineral oils. They may be beneficial for babies, especially those with dry skin and atopic dermatitis
- *Baby powders*: Best avoided in the newborn period; excessive use can block sweat duct pores and lead to miliaria,[2,10] accidental inhalation is another hazard.[10]
- *Baby shampoos*: These are soaps or synthetic detergents especially formulated for cleaning the hair, removal of crusts and scales in infantile seborrheic dermatitis. They usually contain both cleansing agents and lather enhancers.[11]

ROLE OF EMOLLIENTS IN NEONATAL AND INFANTILE SKIN CARE

Although emollients have a generalized role of keeping the skin moist and smooth by trapping water in the epidermis, there are a few conditions where use of emollients is of added benefit playing a precise role in their management or prevention. A few such conditions are given below:
- *Care of the diaper area*: Apart from the frequent change of napkins and keeping the skin airy and dry, emollients (e.g., petroleum, zinc oxide paste) play an important role in the removal of sticky stools and thus prevent the occurrence of diaper dermatitis. However, once diaper dermatitis has set in anti-inflammatory agents may be needed (1% hydrocortisone) along with treatment of the cause (e.g., infection). Recent reports suggest shampoo-clay (Bentonite) may be effective in the treatment of diaper rash.[12]
- *Prevention and/or treatment of atopic dermatitis*: The role of emollients as a treatment modality for atopic dermatitis is well known; interestingly there are few reports which suggest neonatal use of emollients may play a role even in the prevention of atopic dermatitis in the future.[5]
- *Different types of ichthyotic/xerotic skin conditions*.

EMOLLIENTS AVAILABLE IN THE INDIAN MARKET

Currently, the Indian market is flooded with a wide variety of emollients/moisturizers (Table 2) and so each parent has a wide gamut of choices from which they can select the most appropriate. Proper physician advice should always be sought to choose the most suitable product. Minimal use of topical agents in the newborn period is advised.

Table 2: Common emollients/moisturizers available in India

Name of the moisturizers	Chief ingredients
Physiogel lotion (hypoallergenic)	Phospholipids, triglycerides, squalene, cholestrol, ceramides
Physiogel cream (hypoallergenic)	Phospholipids, triglycerides, squalene, cholestrol, ceramides
Cetaphil moisturizing cream/lotion	Water, glycerin, polyethylene glycol (PEG)-2 stearate, cetearyl alcohol, shea butter, dimethicone, stearyl alcohol, etc.
Atopiclair cream/lotion	Vitamin E, vitamin C, glycyrrhetinic acid, hyaluronic acid, shea butter, telmesteine, etc.
Elovera moisturizing cream/lotion	Aloe vera, vitamin E, purified water, white soft paraffin, glycerin, cetyl alcohol, stearic acid, etc.
Emolene cream	Lecithin, propylene glycol, dimethicone, urea, etc.
Episoft lotion	Cetyl alcohol, cetostearyl alcohol, butylene glycol, sodium lauryl sulfate, etc.
Hemont	White soft paraffin, light liquid paraffin, aloe vera extract, lactic acid, urea (2%), squalene, lanolin, etc.
Luciara	Purified water, glycerin, lactic acid, cetostearyl alcohol, sodium lactate, petroleum jelly, etc.
Taiyu silk cream	Aloe vera, shea butter, glycerin, etc.
Venusia/Venusia max	Aloe vera, propylene glycol, wax, squalene, glycerin, cetyl alcohol, stearic acid, dimethicone, vitamin E, etc.
Amylac cream	Ammonium lactate (12%)
Oilatum cream	Liquid paraffin (petrolatum), white soft paraffin
Oilatum lotion	Liquid paraffin (petrolatum), white soft paraffin
Oilatum emollient	Light liquid paraffin (63.4% w/w), isopropyl plamitate, isopropyl alcohol
Cotaryl	Lactic acid (6%), urea (12%), glycine, ammonium chloride, etc.

REFERENCES

1. Sarkar R, Basu S, Agarwal RK, et al. Skin care for the newborn. Indian Pediatr. 2010;47(7): 593-8.
2. Dhar S. Newborn skin care revisited. Indian J Dermatol. 2007;52:1-4.
3. Basu S, Gupta P. Care of the normal newborn. In: Gupta P (Ed). Essential Pediatric Nursing. New Delhi: CBS Publishers and Distributors; 2007. pp. 217-26.
4. Pasricha JS, Gupta R, Gupta SK. Contact hypersensitivity to mustard khal and mustard oil. Indian J Dermatol Venereol Leprol. 1975;51:108-10.
5. Horimukai K, Morita K, Narita M, et al. Application of moisturizer to neonates prevent development of atopic dermatitis. J Allergy Clin Immunol. 2014;134(4):824-30.
6. Hsu SP. Treatment principles. In: Arndt KA, Hsu JT (Eds). Manual of Dermatologic Therapeutics. USA: Lippincott Williams & Wilkins; 2007. pp. 267-72.
7. Danby SG, AlEnezi T, Sultan A, et al. Effect of olive and sunflower seed oil on the adult skin barrier: implications for neonatal skin care. Pediatr Dermatol. 2013;30(1):42-50.
8. Darmstadt GL, Saha SK, Ahmed AS, et al. Effect of skin barrier therapy on neonatal mortality rates in preterm infants in Bangladesh: a randomized, controlled, clinical trial. Pediatrics. 2008;121(3):522-9.
9. Lavender T, Bedwell C, O'Brien E, et al. Infant skin-cleansing product versus water: a pilot randomized, assessor-blinded controlled trial. BMC Pediatr. 2011;11:35.
10. Mofensin HC, Greenshen J, Di Tamasso A, et al. Baby powder--a hazard! Pediatrics. 1981;68(2):265-6.
11. Spoor HJ. Shampoos. Cutis. 1973;12:671-2.
12. Hajbaghery MA, Mahmoudi M, Mashaiekhi M. Shampoo-clay heals diaper rash faster than *Calendula officinalis*. Nurs Midwifery Stud. 2014;3(2):e14180.

CHAPTER 12

Moisturizers and Barrier Creams in Hand Eczema

Rahul Arora, Pallavi Ailawadi

INTRODUCTION

Hand eczema (HE), also called hand dermatitis, is an inflammation of the skin of the hands but rarely may extend to involve the feet. Typical clinical signs are redness, infiltration of the skin, scaling, edema, vesicles, areas of hyperkeratosis, cracks (fissures), and erosions. A wide range of external and internal factors acting singly or in combination, are responsible for such changes. It is usually a manifestation of irritant contact dermatitis, however allergic exacerbation of the disease is well known. The role of barrier defect in the pathogenesis of HE has been an important topic of research which has both etiological and therapeutic implications. A good skin barrier is believed to help preserving the moisture of the skin along with helping avoid the exposure to both irritants and allergens. As a large number of acute eczema progress into chronicity with episodic flares and remissions, importance of skin care and moisturization becomes an important adjuvant treatment to specific measures in long-term management of HE.[1]

EPIDEMIOLOGY AND CLINICAL PATTERNS OF HAND ECZEMA

Incidence and Prevalence

The prevalence of HE has been studied worldwide and appears to be omnipresent. It is common, with a point prevalence of 4% among adults in the general population.[2] In a Swedish epidemiological study by Meding, et al. constituting of 20,000 individuals between ages 20 and 65 years, the prevalence of HE occasionally during the study year was found to be 11%. The incidence of occupational HE is much more and severe with a much higher incidence among certain occupations, such as hairdressing, health care workers and factory workers. Being dermatologists, we also have a tendency towards frequent washing of hand using disinfectants. Furthermore, HE was found to be almost twice as common in females as in males, with a ratio of 1.9, and was most common in young females.[3]

Clinical Patterns

The earliest clinical description of HE in the 19th century included several morphological variants of HE such as eczema solare, rubrum, impetiginoides, squamosum, papulosum, and marginatum. However, the recent classification of HE is based upon etiology, morphology and site of involvement (Table 1), but no single classification is completely satisfactory. Various clinical patterns described in literature include pompholyx variety, patchy vesiculobullous eczema, hyperkeratotic palmar eczema (Figure 1), recurrent focal palmar peeling, discoid eczema, wear and tear dermatitis and ring dermatitis. Clinically, it may present as symptoms of itch and pain associated with erythema, vesicles, papules, scaling, fissuring and hyperkeratosis. Chronic HE is considered when the duration is of more than 6 months. Histopathology is consistent in all patterns with epidermal spongiosis, acanthosis, parakeratosis, infiltration by lymphocytes, while dermis showing vascular dilatation and lymphocytic infiltration.[2]

ETIOPATHOGENESIS OF HAND ECZEMA: ROLE OF MOISTURIZERS

The multifactorial etiology of HE can be broadly divided into two groups: exogenous and endogenous causes, and it is the exogenous contact irritants that are most commonly blamed for HE. These include soaps, detergents, rubber, vegetables, cutting oils, etc.

Contact allergic dermatitis to exogenous antigen is also an important pathogenetic factor. A study conducted by Meding, et al. found a positive patch test to allergens in 32% cases with nickel and cobalt being most commonly implicated.[3] A similar study by Bajaj, et al. from north India reported a positive patch test in 59% of the study subjects with nickel being the most common allergen.[4]

Amongst the endogenous factors, atopic eczema is the most important, thus implying defect in skin barrier as an integral component in pathogenesis of HE.

Table 1: Classification of hand eczema

Etiology

- Irritant HE
- Allergic HE
- Atopic HE
- Others

Morphology

- Dyshidrotic
- Erythema, desquamation
- Hyperkeratotic/rhagadiform
- Nummular

Site

- Dorsum
- Palm
- Sides of the fingers
- Fingertips
- Finger webs
- Wrists

Other

- Chronic acral dermatitis
- Gut/slaughterhouse eczema
- Patchy papulosquamous eczema

HE, hand eczema.

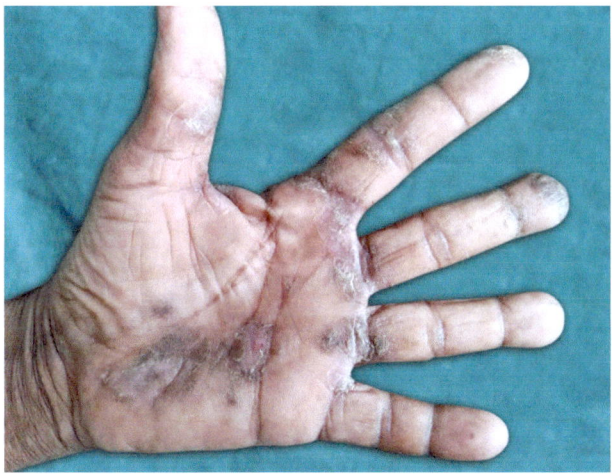

Figure 1: Hyperkeratotic palmar eczema.

Skin Barrier and Hand Eczema

The current literature on the physiological properties, anatomic characteristics, and structural and functional properties of the epidermal barrier of hand skin and its role in pathogenesis of HE is still evolving. However, drawing a correlation with knowledge of normal epidermal barrier function and its responses to alteration in stratum corneum (SC) permeability and damage has helped understanding the pathogenesis of HE.

The components integral to a normal barrier function include claudin, desmoglein, filaggrin, ceramide, proteases, and various scaffolding proteins (involucrin, envoplakin, and periplakin). The main function is to prevent epidermal invasion of allergens and bacteria, and also to prevent water loss. The SC consists of a multicellular vertically stacked layer of cells embedded within a hydrophobic extracellular matrix derived from the secretion of lipid precursors and lipid hydrolases. These hydrolases cleave the precursors to form essential and nonessential fatty acids, cholesterol, and at least 10 different ceramides, which self-organize into multilayered lamellar bilayers with the corneocytes arranged in a water-tight "brick and mortar" pattern, thus maintaining skin hydration.[5] Tight junctions and various scaffolding proteins further help in maintaining skin barrier.

- *Claudins* are a family of proteins that are important components of the tight junctions between corneocytes. This tight junction also blocks access through the skin to various external environmental allergens. Thus, claudin may help in prevention of immune exposure to allergic stimuli.[5]
- *Scaffolding proteins* are required for effective epidermal barrier. Loss of epidermal scaffolding proteins such as involucrin, envoplakin, and periplakin is associated with alterations in epidermal barrier function and altered formation of cornified epidermal envelope.[6]

- *SPINK* is a protein that inhibits serine protease action in the skin. Increased protease activity negatively alters filaggrin and lipid (ceramide) processing thereby decreasing skin barrier function.[2]
- *Filaggrin* is an important protein found in lamellar bodies of stratum granulosum corneocytes. Filaggrin normally assists in cytoskeletal aggregation and formation of the cornified epidermal envelope. Therefore, a filaggrin mutation contributes to a disrupted epidermal barrier, increased water loss, inflammation and exposure to environmental allergens resulting in atopic HE. Detergents cause SC damage by removal of the surface lipid layer and increase transepidermal water loss (TEWL) leading to irritant contact dermatitis.[7]

MOISTURIZERS AND BARRIER CREAMS

The term "moisturizer" is considered more of a marketing term for the consumers who perceive moisturizer as a product to increase water content of skin. However, as dermatologist, we perceive moisturizers as therapeutic agents which can hydrate and improve skin appearance (emollients), create a hydrophobic barrier to decrease TEWL (occlusives) or attract water, thereby increasing epidermal water content (humectants). The details of this classification have been discussed in previous chapters.

"Barrier creams" on the other hand are preparations which can be a cream, ointment or aerosol spray often containing substances which repel water such as silicone, zinc oxide, or dimethicone. This property finds the utility of barrier creams in HE as well as napkin dermatitis. They may also have a property of repelling certain mineral oils, gasoline, lubricants and ink which find its importance in industrial installations for protecting the worker's skin. Barrier creams are often recommended for the prevention of occupational contact dermatitis, but a Cochrane systematic review concluded that there is insufficient evidence that such creams have a long-term protective effect.[8]

Recently, emollients containing skin-related lipids have been introduced. This new generation of emollients is believed to improve the skin barrier dysfunction by being incorporated into the multilayered structure of the intercellular space or in cells of the SC. A good skin barrier helps to avoid the penetration of both allergens and irritants.[9]

The main putative goals in the treatment of HE, therefore may be improvement of the skin barrier function as well as hydration by well-selected emollients.

Mechanism of Action

The details of action of moisturizers in maintaining the barrier function has been well described in the previous chapters. Their main action involves repairing the skin barrier, retaining/increasing water content, reducing TEWL, restoring the lipid barriers' ability to attract, hold and redistribute water, and maintaining skin integrity and appearance. Moisturizers containing collagen and other proteins, i.e., keratin and elastin, claim to rejuvenate the skin by replenishing its essential proteins but their action is still speculative. Moisturizers also act to reduce skin friction and increase skin hydration by providing water directly to the skin from their water phase and by increasing occlusion, measured as a decrease in TEWL.

Moisturizers have little effect on the mechanical properties (i.e., distensibility, hysteresis, and elasticity) of the skin but do increase skin hydration significantly, as shown by an increased skin capacitance.[10]

Formulations and Preparations

Nearly all preparations available in market are a combination of emollients, occlusives, and humectants. Combining occlusives and humectants enhances the water-holding capacity of the skin. Also, the esthetic properties of the moisturizer and the stability of the active ingredients can be influenced by the addition of certain emollients. When glycerol, a humectant, is combined with occlusive agents, there is a synergistic alleviation of dry skin.

Technically, ointments are preferred over creams, because creams may contain potentially sensitizing preservatives and mildly irritating emulsifiers. However, the predominant form of delivery is the cosmetic emulsion with majority being creams (water-in-oil emulsions) and less commonly, lotions (oil-in-water emulsions). Moreover, complicated emulsions (e.g., oil-in-water-in-oil, oleaginous mixtures, serums, gels, sprays, and milks) are formulated to deliver and stabilize some active ingredients. The esthetics vary in accordance with consumer preferences and the desired attributes. They determine the compliance of the patient as well. The precise nature of these formulations is not disclosed and the ingredients are not always listed on the product.[10] Table 2 enlists some of the common formulations available in India.

Table 2: Some hand care products available in India	
Product	Composition
Pharmaceutical product	
Cetaphil® cream	Petrolatum, dimethicone
Venusia Max cream	Propylene glycol, wax, glycerine, cyclomethicone, shea butter
Oilatum cream	White soft paraffin, liquid paraffin, glycerol
Fixderma moisturizing cream	Urea, lactic acid, aloe vera extract, almond oil, vitamin E
OTC Cosmetic hand preparation	
Organic hand and foot care lotion	Glycerine, aloe vera, apricot oil, coconut oil
Neutrogena Norwegian Formula hand cream	Glycerin, dimethicone
Aveeno® moisturizing cream	Shea butter, colloidal oatmeal
Clinique Deep Comfort hand and cuticle cream	Octyldodecyl myristate, cetyl alcohol, stearyl alcohol, dimethicone, glycerin,
Vita Age Aurum regenerating anti spot hand treatment	Hyaluronic acid, stem cells of *Leontopodium alpinum*, vitamins A, C, E and UVA-UVB filters
Vivel Cell Renew Repair + Fortifying hand cream	Aqua, glycerin, mineral oil, acrylates/acrylamide copolymer, polysorbate 85, isohexadecane, cetyl alcohol
Aloe Veda hand and cuticle cream	Almond oil, beeswax, butter
Garnier hand repair	Glycerin

Frequency of Applications

Although a frequent application of emollients and moisturizers is routinely recommended, the data regarding frequency of application is unclear. Warshaw recommended 15 times a day application of the moisturizer in ideal situation; such strategy is bound to be unpopular and impractical. Moreover, there are reports of colonization of *Staphylococcus aureus, Staphylococcus epidermidis, Candida* and *Aspergillus* species. However, application of a moisturizer after every hand wash has proven to improve the skin dryness and roughness caused by frequent hand washing.[2]

Method of Application

Most preparations mention the relevant procedure of application on the product under "HOW TO USE" logo. However, Health and Safety Executive recommends a detailed procedure for hand cream application (Figure 2) which involves a palm to palm application first followed by palm to back of hand with finger over laced, palm to palm with finger interlaced, fingers interlocked, followed by rotational rubbing of thumb in palm, rotational rubbing of fingertips on palm and application on each wrist.[11]

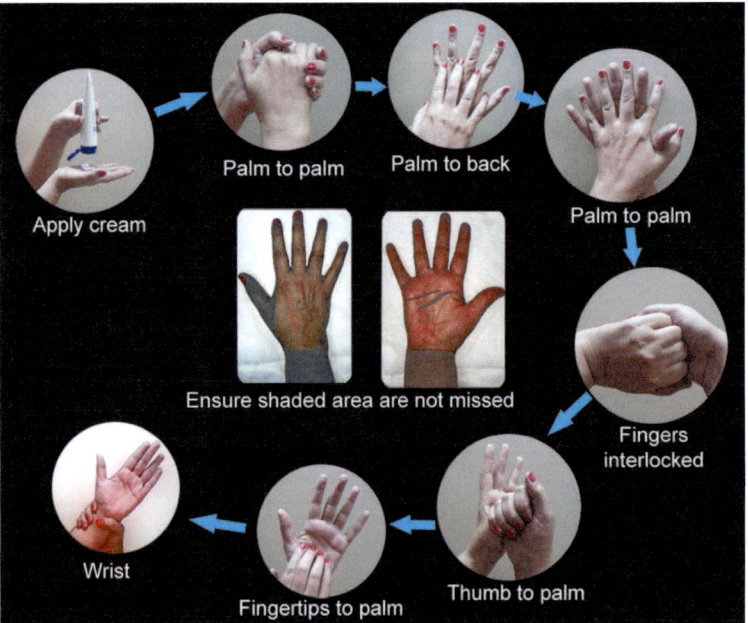

Figure 2: Demonstrating how to apply hand cream.
Courtesy: Dr Rahul Arora (Demonstrating method by Health and Safety Executive, UK: Method of using hand cream, soap, and cleanser)

EVIDENCE OF USE OF MOISTURIZERS AND BARRIER CREAMS IN HAND ECZEMA

Evidence to make recommendations on moisturizers is meager and the preventive effectiveness of moisturizers needs to be established. However, the market is flooded with product categorized under cosmetic hand creams with minimal evidence on their efficacy and which, according to European Union legislation, cannot be recommended for treatment of skin diseases.

In one of the first studies in 1943, a urea-containing moisturizer was found to be superior to a urea-free cream inducing softer, smoother, and even whiter, hands in 225 hospital personnel.[12,13]

Thereafter, the European Dermato-Epidemiology Network (EDEN) hand eczema survey in 2004 found that there were only 11 clinical trials and 1 randomized control trial on use of moisturizers and barrier creams in HE.[14]

Clinical trials related to the subject of skin protective creams can be divided into three main groups:[15] (1) skin protection is effective and addresses issues such as acceptance or the correct application; (2) studies confirming the efficacy of skin protective measures in highly standardized study designs; (3) the third group includes studies reporting (even negative) effects of skin protection.

- Perrenoud, et al. found a protective cream containing aluminum chlorohydrate 5% as active ingredient to be as effective as its vehicle[15]
- Bendt, et al. compared Excipial Protect barrier cream (containing 2% urea and 11% lipid), used 50 hospital nurses and found it to be effective in decreasing the roughness and texture of skin but was comparable to the vehicle[15]
- Goh, et al. compared use of a barrier cream, an after-work emollient and usage of no creams in machinist exposed to cutting fluid dermatitis. There was no significant difference in incidence of cutting fluid dermatitis in the three groups doubting their utility. However, about 50% fewer cases of cutting fluid dermatitis were observed in the group using after-work emollient cream compared with controls[15]
- Held et al. reported an increased response to sodium lauryl sulfate in moisturizer treated arm with a high lipid content moisturizer[15]
- Lodén, et al. compared a barrier-strengthening formulation containing primarily 5% urea with no treatment or bland non-medicated topical applications found an important role of moisturizers in prevention of relapse of eczema[13]
- A comparison of efficacy of barrier creams with skin care products in a sample of 192 dental technicians showed a clear benefit for moisturizers, which were even superior to barrier creams used before and during working hours[15]
- Interestingly, Kutting, et al. evaluated the role of moisturizers and barrier cream in prevention of HE and reported a much better clinical course in participants who used barrier cream before work and moisturizers after work when compared to participants using moisturizer alone or no measures[15]
- Kucharekova, et al. compared an emollient-containing skin-related lipids (ceramide 3, oleic and palmitic acid in a fatty cream base with petrolatum, aqua, paraffin, paraffinum liquidum, glycerin, sorbitan oleate, carnauba, cholesterol, carbomer, tromethamine in unknown ratio; lipid content 63%)

with petrolatum-based emollient as an adjunct in treatment of chronic HE. Although the study concluded that frequent use of emollients in HE is a useful adjunctive treatment with topical corticosteroids, there was no statistical difference in treatment outcomes with the use of lipid-based emollient.[9]

COUNSELING AND EDUCATION

Many dermatologists recommend and counsel the patient regarding the use of gloves or protective wear as a preventive strategy. However, the role of protective gloves is controversial. Although gloves offer protection from irritants (especially during "wet work"), it is also proposed that prolonged occlusion may itself be a risk factor for HE. Moreover, a focus on skin care education and individual counseling has a proven therapeutic role in prevention of relapses.[2]

TREATMENT OF HAND ECZEMA

Hand eczema follows a relapsing and remitting course and remains a challenge for both the patient and the treating dermatologist. Although avoidance of irritants and allergens remains the most obvious and the most common treatment advice, it also happens to be the most difficult task. Maintenance of barrier function and prevention of disruption remains the underlying principle of management. Various lifestyle modifications may help in achieving the same and further potentiate the good clinical outcomes. These are enlisted in Box 1.

Topical corticosteroids form the mainline therapy combined with emollients and oral antihistamines. Other topical modalities include tar preparations, salicylic acid, dithranol, bexarotene, topical calcineurin inhibitors, topical vitamin D analogs, topical antibiotics, intradermal botulinum toxin, and iontophoresis. Oral steroids in short tapering course, oral immunosuppressive therapy with cyclosporine, methotrexate or azathioprine, oral retinoids may be used in severe recalcitrant cases.[2]

Box 1: Lifestyle modifications and hand care practices to prevent hand eczema

- Use gloves in wet work environment
- Gloves must be used for as long a time as necessary but for as short a time as possible
- Use cotton gloves underneath protective gloves
- Wash hands in cool water and dry them well
- Alcohol-based disinfectants should be used instead of soap when the hands are not visibly dirty
- Do not wear rings at work
- Use a moisturizer with high amount of fat and no perfume
- The moisturizer must be applied on the whole hand, including the fingers and the back of the hand
- Moisturizing should be repeated many times in a day, ideally 15 times a day
- Moisturizing should be done immediately after wet work, shower to "lock in" the moisture
- For intensive therapy, generous amount of emollient can be applied at night under occlusion (cotton gloves)
- Try not to use hot water and decrease exposure to water to less than 15 minutes at a time, if possible.

CONCLUSION

There are very few reliable studies to inform clinical practice with regard to role of moisturizers and barrier cream in HE, especially in the long-term management. Until such data are forthcoming, an unregulated plethora of cosmeceutical product may continue to prosper amongst the consumers as well as the physicians, many of which will be ineffective or even harmful. There is an utmost requirement to conduct high-quality randomized controlled trials (RCTs) of people with HE, comparing commonly used simple preparations with simple and distinct outcome measures.

REFERENCES

1. Coenraads PJ. Hand eczema. N Engl J Med. 2012;367(19):1829-37.
2. Agarwal US, Besarwal RK, Gupta R, et al. Hand eczema. Indian J Dermatol. 2014;59(3): 213-24.
3. Meding B, Swanbeck G. Prevalence of hand eczema in an industrial city. Br J Dermatol. 1987;116(5):627-34.
4. Bajaj AK, Saraswat A, Mukhija G, et al. Patch testing experience with 1000 patients. Indian J Dermatol Venereol Leprol. 2007;73(5):313-8.
5. Elias PM, Schmuth M. Abnormal skin barrier in the etiopathogenesis of atopic dermatitis. Curr Allergy Asthma Rep. 2009;9(4):265-72.
6. Sevilla LM, Nachat R, Groot KR, et al. Mice deficient in involucrin, envoplakin, and periplakin have a defective epidermal barrier. J Cell Biol. 2007;179(7):1599-612.
7. Morar N, Edster P, Street T, et al. Fine mapping of susceptibility genes for atopic dermatitis in the epidermal differentiation complex on chromosome 1q21. Br J Dermatol. 2007;157:3.
8. Bauer A, Schmitt J, Bennett C, et al. Interventions for preventing occupational irritant hand dermatitis. Cochrane Database Syst Rev. 2010;(6):CD004414.
9. Kucharekova M, van de Kerkhof PC, van der Valk PG. A randomized comparison of emollient containing skin-related lipids with a petrolatum-based emollient as adjunct in the treatment of chronic hand dermatitis. Contact Dermatitis. 2003;48(6):293-9.
10. Kraft JN, Lynde CW. Moisturizers: what they are and a practical approach to product selection. Skin Therapy Lett. 2005;10(5):1-8.
11. Health and Safety Executive, UK. Skin Care: Method of using hand cream, soap, and cleanser. [online] Available at www.hse.gov.uk/skin/posters/skinmethod.pdf. [Accessed June, 2015].
12. Lodén M, Wirén K, Smerud KT, et al. The effect of a corticosteroid cream and a barrier-strengthening moisturizer in hand eczema. A double-blind, randomized, prospective, parallel group clinical trial. J Eur Acad Dermatol Venereol. 2012;26(5):597-601.
13. Lodén M, Wirén K, Smerud K, et al. Treatment with a barrier-strengthening moisturizer prevents relapse of hand-eczema. An open, randomized, prospective, parallel group study. Acta Derm Venereol. 2010;90(6):602-6.
14. Van Coevorden AM, Coenraads PJ, Svensson A, et al. Overview of studies of treatments for hand eczema—the EDEN hand eczema survey. Br J Dermatol. 2004;151(2):446-51.
15. Kutting B, Baumeister T, Weistenhofer W. Effectiveness of skin protection measures in prevention of occupational hand eczema: results of a prospective randomized controlled trial over a follow-up period of 1 year. Br J Dermatol. 2010;162(1):362-70.

CHAPTER 13

Moisturizing Different Racial Skin Types

Michelle Rodrigues

INTRODUCTION

The term "skin of color" was coined in North America and refers to those with non-Caucasian skin types. It includes those with Fitzpatrick skin phototypes III–VI and therefore encompasses many heterogeneous ethnic and cultural groups around the world including people from East Asia, South Asia, Africa, Latin America and the Middle East as well as many indigenous Oceanic and genetically admixed populations. In many western countries around the world including the United States (US) of America, the United Kingdom and Australia, the number of people with skin of color is continually increasing. In fact, the US census indicates that by the year 2056, over half of the US population will be non-Caucasian.[1]

Skin of color is structurally, functionally and esthetically different to white skin. Those with skin of color have an increased prevalence of certain skin conditions and unique reactions to cutaneous stimuli, injury and skin-directed therapy. Such differences must be fully understood and appreciated in order to choose the correct emollient for different patient populations and in different clinical scenarios. Failing to address these differences can result in under-treatment, non-compliance and unnecessary complications.

Emollients are designed to improve texture, appearance and feel of the skin and to reduce itching and irritation. They are the mainstay of treatment and maintenance of atopic dermatitis (AD) and other conditions causing pruritus. In order to be effective, emollients must decrease transepidermal water loss (TEWL), make the skin feel smooth and soft (called "emolliency") and protect the skin from harmful stimuli. A stratum corneum containing approximately 30% water will exhibit the softness and pliability of normal stratum corneum. Studies reveal that those with skin of color aspire for smooth skin and dry skin, uneven skin tone and acne are among the main skin complaints for skin of color patients.[2] Therefore, selecting the correct emollient for these patients is critical.

STRUCTURAL AND FUNCTIONAL DIFFERENCES IN SKIN OF COLOR

There are many biological differences in the skin and hair of those with skin of color. The stratum corneum, ceramide concentration, melanosome number and size, collagen, elastin, glycoproteins and blood vessel composition are just some of the things that are different in skin of color. These factors account for the differences seen in the skin texture, feel, predilection for certain dermatologic conditions and response to trauma demonstrated in this group.

Though the dermis, blood vessels and cutaneous appendages are different in white skin and skin of color, only factors directly relevant to emollient use will be discussed here.

The Stratum Corneum, Corneocytes and Lipids

The stratum corneum is the outermost layer of the skin and is critical for barrier function. Corneocytes (containing keratin and filaggrin) are embedded in a matrix of lipid-enriched membranes. Lipids (such as ceramides and cholesterol) fill the intercellular spaces between corneocytes, which provide the permeability barrier of the skin.

Although the stratum corneum thickness and corneocyte size is approximately the same in black and white skin, the stratum corneum of black skin has more layers and is more compact and cohesive with greater intercellular lipid content compared with white skin. This has been demonstrated in a study in which those with black skin required a greater number of tape strippings to remove the stratum corneum.[3]

Despite the fact that black skin has more lipid content and layers in the stratum corneum, ceramide concentration in the stratum corneum is lowest in blacks, followed by whites, Hispanics and Asians.[4] Ceramide levels are inversely proportional to TEWL and directly related to water content.[5] Lower ceramide levels and increased TEWL give rise to drier (xerosis), itchier skin (Figure 1).

Studies on corneocyte desquamation have revealed variable results suggesting that this may vary by anatomical site rather than by race, as it does in Caucasian skin. Racial differences in corneocyte surface area and skin irritation have been studied but a paucity of well-designed studies has led to inconsistent findings. Further studies are required to obtain more conclusive data.

Transepidermal Water Loss

Study findings on TEWL in different skin types are variable. A few studies have revealed higher TEWL in black and Asian skins while others failed to demonstrate any difference between skin types. The inconsistencies may be due to many factors including variation in anatomical sites studied.

Thus, while some have concluded that more darkly pigmented skin demonstrates superior epidermal barrier function and faster recovery from barrier damage,[6] others have suggested that the higher TEWL in black skin suggests a more compromised epidermal barrier function and increased susceptibility to irritants.

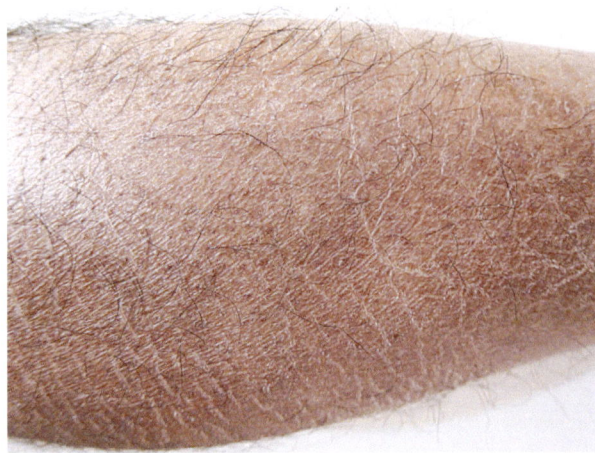

Figure 1: Xerosis.

Skin pH

The skin's natural pH is approximately 5 and when maintained, this pH ensures optimal barrier function and moisturization and results in less scaling on the skin. In addition, this natural pH provides a hospitable milieu for normal skin flora.

Difference in stratum corneum pH between different populations has been explored with variable results. Some studies suggested no difference while others cite a lower pH in those with skin phototype VI. Clearly, more work needs to be done in this area to establish differences in pH between racial groups and anatomical sites.

DIFFERENCE IN DISEASE PREVALENCE, PRESENTATION AND COMPLICATIONS

Atopic Dermatitis

Several studies have revealed an increase in the prevalence of AD among blacks and Asian/Pacific Islanders when compared with Caucasians.[7] Black and/or Asian children in England and the US may have an increased prevalence of AD.[8] The prevalence of AD in northern Europe, the US, Japan and southeastern Nigeria is 15.6, 17.2, 21 and 8.5%, respectively. In an Australian study,[7] the prevalence of AD in Caucasian and Chinese children born in Melbourne was 21 and 44%, respectively. Similar socioeconomic backgrounds in these groups suggest genetic influences do play a role in the prevalence of AD.

Furthermore, the filaggrin-2 mutation variations in AD seen in African-American patients confer a more persistent disease course.[9] Those with skin of color are more likely to have subclinical erythema and a follicular pattern to their eczema (Figures 2A and B), making it less likely to be diagnosed and treated early. Delayed diagnosis and increased severity of eczema in this group makes post-inflammatory hyper- and hypopigmentation more likely, more severe and more prolonged.

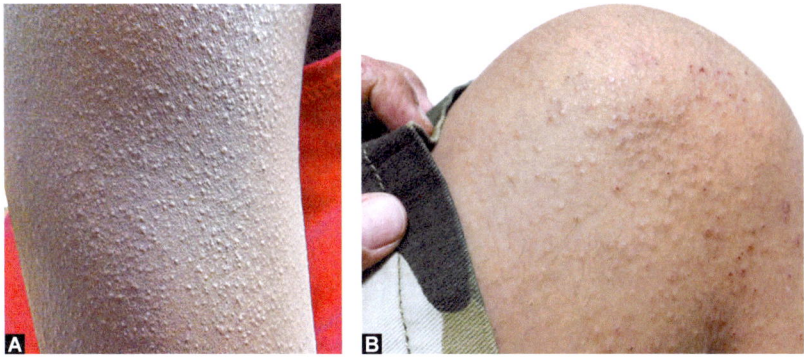

Figure 2: A, Follicular eczma in Fitzpatrik type 6 skin; **B,** Follicular eczema in Fitzpatrick type 4 skin.

Lower ceramide concentrations, possible increased TEWL and genetic susceptibility to more severe eczema make moisturizing skin of color vital. Emollients improve the appearance and symptoms of dry skin associated with eczema and reduce the requirement for topical steroid.[10] The stratum corneum is rehydrated, TEWL is decreased and corneocytes swell to restore the epidermal barrier with emollient use. This results in decreased dryness, itch and irritation of the skin.

Xerosis

Xerosis (dry skin) can lead to whitish coloring and reduced shininess of the skin known as "ashiness" or "ashy skin" in those with skin of color (Figure 3A). Xerosis may be associated with environmental factors including seasonal changes or use of soap. It may also be associated with biological factors including lower ceramide concentration, inefficient corneocyte desquamation and lower expression of serine proteases and cathepsins,[11] all of which are noted in those with skin of color.

While "ashiness" is not a dermatological condition as such, it is one that is cosmetically concerning for many with skin of color. Smoothening skin scale on the stratum corneum can decrease an ashy skin appearance. The ability of an emollient to achieve this is called "emolliency" (Figure 3B). Emolliency results from the temporary filling of spaces between the desquamating skin scales.

Acne

While nodulocystic acne is thought to be less common in skin of color, comedonal acne is more common in this group (Figure 4). Despite the clinical appearance, studies reveal those with black skin have more intense inflammation in acneiform lesions histologically than those with white skin. Interestingly, this group's chief complaint is often "brown marks" or "blemishes" rather than "pimples" or "acne". Furthermore, cosmetically displeasing scarring and hyperpigmentation secondary to acne is more common, more intense and more difficult to treat in this group.

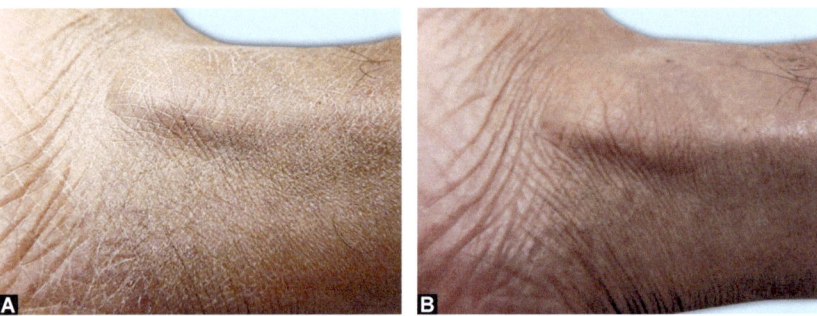

Figure 3: Ashy skin before **(A)** and after **(B)** application of emollient.

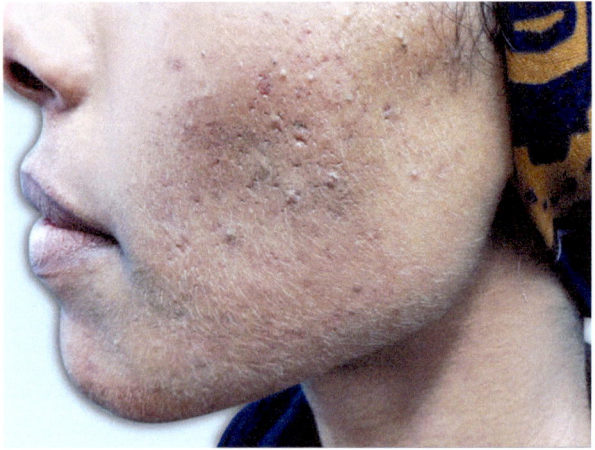

Figure 4: Comedonal acne in Fitzpatrick type 6 skin.

Pomade acne (comedonal acne of the forehead) is more common in skin of color and results from using certain hair care products. Various types of oils, e.g., mineral, nut and olive are the most common culprits and are often employed to manage and style textured hair.

All occlusive emollients (described below) should be discontinued and those that are non-comedogenic should be selected for patients with acne or seborrhea. Use of silicone-based hair care products should also be encouraged to avoid pomade acne.

SPECIAL CONSIDERATIONS IN EMOLLIENT SELECTION FOR SKIN OF COLOR

In order to be used regularly, emollients need to be easy to access, affordable, esthetically pleasing and transparent when applied on skin of color. Providing sample sizes of emollients are a good way of facilitating a pretreatment trial and increasing compliance. Samples enable the patient to determine which product they prefer and are most likely to use.

Types of Emollients

Three main types of emollients are available to rehydrate the stratum corneum—(1) occlusive agents, (2) humectants and (3) hydrophilic matrices. Each of these boasts advantages but their disadvantages must also be carefully considered. Combinations of ingredients from different categories are usually used to achieve different consistencies and esthetics.

1. *Occlusive agents* are most commonly used in those with skin of color as they decrease scales, and thus eliminate ashiness. Many emollients marketed for skin of color contain highly occlusive agents like shea, cocoa butter, and mineral oil. While occlusive agents are greasy and thick, they are the most effective agents in decreasing water loss. They provide a water-impermeable coating over the stratum corneum to create an artificial barrier. Examples of occlusive agents include petrolatum and mineral oil. It should be noted, as mentioned above, that those with a history of acne or folliculitis should avoid occlusive emollients.
2. *Humectants* absorb water from the dermis into the dehydrated epidermis. Those with skin of color are less likely to use humectants as they can increase the appearance of ashy skin if the concentration of occlusive ingredients is not high enough. Furthermore, humectants can increase water loss if the skin barrier is defective. Examples of humectants include glycerin and urea.
3. *Hydrophilic matrix* emollients physically prevent water from evaporating from the damaged stratum corneum. Depending on the proteins being used, these may form an invisible film over the skin making it esthetically pleasing for those with skin of color. Examples include colloidal oatmeal and synthetic proteins.

Studies demonstrate that newer ceramide-containing emollients improve itching and dryness in AD[12] and these may be useful for some patients with skin of color in whom ceramide concentration are low. The formulation of the emollient is also critical when considering aesthetics and function. Day creams usually contain an occlusive ingredient with water in a lotion formula, while night creams are usually thicker and more moisturizing. Oil-free formulations will usually substitute mineral oil with dimethicone and should be used in those with acne or seborrhea.

Emollient-Containing Sunscreen

A plethora of emollient-containing sunscreens are available for consumers but are more commonly marketed for those with fairer skin types. Furthermore, many of these products (especially titanium-based products) leave a chalky white hue on the skin when used in those with skin of color.

While those with black skin have intrinsic protection (melanin) against DNA damage caused by ultraviolet light, there are many compelling reasons for those with skin of color to use an emollient-containing sunscreen on a daily basis. Firstly, regular use of sunscreen reduces the risk of developing dyschromias. Dyschromias are considered one of the visible signs of aging in this patient group and is a very common reason for those with skin of color to consult with a dermatologist. Secondly, sunscreen also increases the effectiveness of hydroquinone therapy, which is the gold standard for treatment of hyperpigmented dermatoses such as melasma and post-inflammatory hyperpigmentation. Finally, but importantly, regular sunscreen prevents photoaging. This is another good reason for those with skin of color to maintain a sun-protection routine. While the development of ultraviolet light-induced skin cancers is not common in this group of patients, it has been reported and is another good reason for application of sunscreen.

For the reasons mentioned above, those with skin of color should be encouraged to use a good quality, broad-spectrum, emollient-containing sunscreen. In order to increase compliance, those with skin of color can be encouraged to wear newer physical blockers that are micronized. These blend into the skin more readily than titanium-based products and are, therefore, more aesthetically acceptable for pigmented skin. Chemical sunscreens are of course, another option for pigmented skin. Using an emollient-containing sunscreen will not only decrease ashiness of the skin and make it appear smoother and more luminous but will also prevent the development of dyschromias and skin cancers in the future.

CONCLUSION

Successfully moisturizing different racial skin types require an understanding of the structural and functional differences in skin of color. It also requires an appreciation for the main concerns, disease prevalence and clinical nuances in this diverse group of patients. The correct type and form of emollient can then be selected to meet the individual patient's needs and expectations.

REFERENCES

1. US Census Bureau. Population projections of the US by age, sex, race and Hispanic origin: 1995-2050. Current population report: 25-1130. Washington DC: US Government Press; 2002.
2. El-Essawi D, Musial JL, Hammad A, et al. A survey of skin disease and skin-related issues in Arab Americans. J Am Acad Dermatol. 2007;56(6):933-8.
3. Weigand DA, Haygood C, Gaylor JR. Cell layers and density of Negro and Caucasian stratum corneum. J Invest Dermatol. 1974;62(6):563-8.
4. Badreshia-Bansal S, Taylor SC. The structure and function of skin of color. In: Kelly PA, Kelly AP, Taylor SC (Eds). Dermatology for Skin of Color. New York: McGraw-Hill: 2009. pp. 71-7.
5. Sugino K, Imokawa G, Maibach HI. Ethnic differences of stratum corneum lipid in relation to stratum corneum function. J Invest Dermatol. 1993;100:597.
6. Gunathilake R, Schurer NY, Shoo BA, et al. pH-regulated mechanisms account for pigment-type differences in epidermal barrier function. J Invest Dermatol. 2009;129(7):1719-29.
7. Mar A, Tam M, Jolley D, et al. The cumulative incidence of atopic dermatitis in the first 12 months among Chinese, Vietnamese and Caucasian infants born in Melbourne, Australia. J Am Acad Dermatol. 1999;40(4):597-602.
8. Zar HJ, Ehrlich RI, Workman L, et al. The changing prevalence of asthma, allergic rhinitis and atopic eczema in African adolescents from 1995 to 2002. Pediatr Allergy Immunol. 2007;18(7):560-5.
9. Margolis DJ, Gupta J, Apter AJ, et al. Filaggrin-2 variation is associated with more persistent atopic dermatitis in African American subjects. J Allergy Clin Immunol. 2014;133(3):784-9.
10. Williams HC. Clinical practice. Atopic dermatitis. N Engl J Med. 2005;352(22):2314-24.
11. Chen N, Seiberg M, Lin CB. Cathepsin L2 levels inversely correlate with skin color. J Invest Dermatol. 2006;126(10):2345-7.
12. Lynde CW, Andriessen A. A cohort study on a ceramide-containing cleanser and moisturizer used for atopic dermatitis. Cutis. 2014;93(4):207-13.

CHAPTER 14

Moisturizers for Indian Skin: Geographical, Cultural, and Regional Variations

Ishad Aggarwal, Sahil Mrigpuri

INTRODUCTION

In today's scenario, the term "moisturizer" is not just restricted to a bland oleaginous substance that is rubbed on the skin to provide moisture. Driven by the boom in cosmetic industry, moisturizers have transformed from simple hydrating creams to luxurious therapeutic and antiaging products, rampantly advertised over the media, sold over the counters and purchased all across the nation, by all strata of society.

How often are dermatologists queried by their patients regarding the best moisturizer to use amongst the array of products available? Although such a decision may have been made arbitrarily in the past, however, as more scientific information on skin care formulations continues to emerge, we dermatologists need to give more thought to not just the moisturizer formulations and their differences, but a host of patient factors too. The aim of this chapter is to highlight some important factors an Indian dermatologist must consider before prescribing a moisturizer, because of the unique racial, social and geographical variations seen in our diverse country.

CHOOSING THE RIGHT MOISTURIZER

While prescribing a moisturizer, one must assess a lot of factors. Some of these factors are intrinsic to the skin of the patient presenting to the treating dermatologist, while some are dependent upon the environment the patient might be exposed to. Hence, all these factors must be considered in concert with each other and a patient must be assessed as a whole.

FACTORS INTRINSIC TO INDIAN SKIN

The modern Indian population is a polygenetic amalgamation of various ethnicities and racial subtypes. Broadly speaking, the fascinating mix that we see in India is of following major types:
- *Nordics or the Indo-Aryans*: They are predominantly located in the northern and Central India, and have *Caucasoid* features.

- *Negritos*: The Negritos or the Brachycephalics are the earliest people to have come to India and are broad headed and have African descent. They are mainly seen in the islands of Andaman and Nicobar and some hill tribes of southern part of mainland of India.
- *Pro-Australoids*: These groups were the next to come to India after the Negritos. These people have long heads and low foreheads and prominent eye ridges, thick jaws and small chins. Their skin is brown, with wavy hair luxuriously distributed over their bodies. The Austrics of India represent a race of medium height, dark complexion with long heads and rather flat noses but otherwise of regular features. Now these people are found in some parts of South India, Myanmar and the islands of Southeast Asia. Their languages have survived in the central and eastern India.
- *Dravidians*: The Dravidians are people of South India and have features which are Australoid, paleo-Mediterranean and oriental Mediterranean.
- *Mongoloids*: These are people found in the northeastern and some hilly tribes of North India. They have fair complexion, high cheekbones and oblique eyes.
- *Miscellaneous*: Some of the Indian population is also a mix of Alpenoids and Armenians, and are mainly concentrated in Kashmir, western Gujarat, Rajasthan and Maharashtra, and mainly consist of the Parsis and Kodavas.

In this day and age, due to hypermobility of people all across the country and worldwide, we as dermatologists see people belonging to all ethnicities in any part of the country. Knowing the subtle racial differences in skin composition may help a dermatologist choose the right moisturizer for his patient.

RACIAL DIFFERENCES IN VARIOUS SKIN TYPES

Most of the studies that have been conducted on skin's ability to retain moisture were performed on the Caucasian skin. However, recently although in a small sample size, researchers have been able to elucidate racial differences in some important parameters that govern the skin's ability to retain moisture. The factors that were studied were, transepidermal water loss (TEWL), water content, ceramide levels and skin reactivity. Needless to say that in context of the present book, these factors are really important when one needs to choose a moisturizer formulation.[1]

- *Transepidermal water loss*: Transepidermal water loss is the amount of water vapor lost from skin when there is no sweat gland activity.[2] Although there are conflicting reports from various researchers regarding racial differences in this skin parameter, however, on interpretation of all available data, it becomes apparent that some differences do exist. It has been seen that TEWL is higher in African-American skin compared to Caucasian skin. Kompaore, et al. have reported that after removing upper stratum corneum, Asian skin type (Mongoloid skin) has maximum permeability compared to Blacks and Caucasians. These factors highlight the ability of various skin types to withstand exogenous insults, maintain moisture and recover after damage has been done.[3,4]

- *Ceramides*: Ceramides are waxy lipids composed of sphingosine and fatty acids. They act in concert with cholesterol and are essential for barrier function of the epidermis. Sugino, Imokawa and Maibach found that ceramide levels were inversely correlated with TEWL and directly proportional to water content of the skin.[5] It was seen that Blacks had lowest levels of ceramide in their skin, followed by whites and Hispanics and Asians.
- *Water content*: Water content or level of hydration of skin has been assessed in various racial skin types using galvanic current, capacitance, and resistance.[6] It is seen that dry skin has maximum resistance and least conductance of current. Therefore, it was found that skin of Blacks has less water content than skin of Caucasians. One study demonstrated that Asian skin has more hydration than Caucasian and Black skins.[5]
- *pH*: The pH of African skin has been found to be lower than Caucasian skin.
- *Corneocyte shedding*: Although still a matter of significant debate, some workers have found increased corneocyte shedding in Black skin.
- *Skin irritability*: Taking vascular response as a marker of skin irritability, it has been found that Negroid skin is most predisposed to irritability by irritants, and therefore easily susceptible to loss of barrier function.[7] Mongoloid skin is least susceptible to skin irritability.

Although none of the studies of biochemical and physiological properties of ethnic skin has been performed on the Indian ethnic groups, however, basic idea of such variations in above mentioned skin types and their resemblance to Indian ethnic groups must be borne in mind while prescribing a moisturizer to Indian patients.

CULTURAL HABITS AND LIFESTYLE

Culturally, modern India stands at crossroads between fading traditional practices and rising western trends. There are a lot of cultural practices varying from region to region and indigenous to particular areas, which may affect the hydration of skin, and therefore affect the choice of moisturizing formulation. Thus clues must be sought from history and some of them may even lie scattered on cutaneous examination.

Application of various kinds of oils on the body is a very common practice which may make skin comedogenic, and hence preclude the usage of an occlusive moisturizer. Similarly, applications of honey, milk, cream and curd is common among Indian women. Fuller's earth or multani mitti applied as a mud pack on face in India causes dryness of skin.

However, insult to skin is not just a traditional phenomenon. With increasing demand for beauty, there is a rampant usage of fairness creams and beauty treatments in India. There are a variety of products sold over the counter. A history and knowledge of key ingredients of such cosmetic products is vital to dermatologists. These products may cause overhydration of skin and in some cases may even strip the stratum corneum of essential lipids and compromise the barrier function. Similarly, a meticulous record of parlor activities may be sought to understand the true nature of exposure that skin of patient routinely undergoes. It is also imperative that a patient presenting with need of a moisturizer also be asked about the nature of their job in order to prescribe a moisturizer that is compatible with ergonomics. Certain practices like over cleansing of skin, usage of retinoid-containing formulations in fairness creams should in fact be discouraged as they may cause iatrogenic xerosis of skin.

History of hypersensitivity, contact sensitization, contact dermatitis should also be obtained in order to provide a safe moisturizer as the patient may develop a break in integrity of skin due to component of the moisturizer prescribed.[8]

Skin being the largest surface of body bears direct insult due to various human activities. An astute dermatologist should be aware of common cultural practices pertaining to skin and their impact on it.

GEOGRAPHICAL AND GEOCLIMATIC VARIATIONS IN INDIA

India experiences large variations in climate from region to region. India can be divided into four major types of climatic groups. Seasonal variations must be borne into mind by a dermatologist while choosing a moisturizer.

1. *Tropical wet/dry humid group*: Temperature never goes below 18°C, the summers are very hot and precipitation is very high. The western ghats, Malabar peninsular plateau region, southern parts of Assam and eastern Tamil Nadu fall in this region.
2. *Subtropical humid group*: The winter climate goes below 18°C. Himalayan foothills, Punjab, Haryana, northern parts of West Bengal, Uttar Pradesh and Bihar fall in this zone.
3. *Mountain regions*: Northern states of Himachal Pradesh, Kashmir, Uttarakhand, northeastern States of Sikkim and Arunachal Pradesh. The winters are subzero and dry. Summers are pleasant and monsoons receive moderate precipitation.
4. *Tropical arid/subtropical arid zone*: These are regions where evaporation of skin is more than moisture of air and are predominated by dry weather throughout the year.

It is important to know these geographical variations, since we know that winters have drying effect on skin. Some of the moisturizing formulations may be too sticky and greasy for a warm humid climate, while others may not suffice in extreme cold and arid weathers.

AYURVEDA AND COMPLIMENTARY THERAPIES

Ayurvedic skin care and moisturizers were derived from medicinal practices that began over 5,000 years ago in India. Ayurvedic medicine and healing practices are based on Indian philosophical, psychological, conventional, and medicinal understandings.

Most of the skin care products contain the following herbs—aloe vera, almond, avocado, carrot, castor, clay, cocoa, coconut oil, cornmeal, cucumber, cutch tree, emu oil, *Ginkgo biloba*, ginseng, grape seed oil, ground almond and walnut shell, horse chestnut, witch hazel and honey.

Egg Oil

Egg oil has many applications in skin care and can be used as an excipient/carrier in a variety of cosmetic preparations as an emollient, moisturizer, antioxidant, penetration enhancer, occlusive skin conditioner and antibacterial agent. As an occlusive agent, it protects against dehydration without disturbing the pores and is easily incorporated in topical preparations since it forms stable oil-in-water emulsions.

Honey

Honey's natural antioxidant and antimicrobial properties, and ability to absorb and retain moisture have been recognized and used extensively in skin care treatments as they help to protect the skin from the damage from ultraviolet (UV) light and rejuvenate depleted skin.

Shea Butter

Shea butter is derived from the kernel of the shea tree (*Vitellaria paradoxa*). Shea butter is known for its cosmetic properties as a moisturizer and emollient.

Jojoba

Jojoba is used for skin care because it is a natural moisturizer for the skin. Jojoba is actually a liquid wax that becomes solid below room temperature, but is known as oil.

Algae

Polysaccharides derived from algae are natural moisturizers and can be used in cosmetics as humectants.

TYPES OF MOISTURIZERS AND SKIN TYPES

Stratum corneum is a dynamic structure and maintenance of hydration is vital for its functioning. There are various kinds of moisturizers and all of them either provide hydration or repair the hydrating ability of skin.

- *Humectants* are substances that attract water when applied to the skin.[9] In this manner, they theoretically improve hydration of the stratum corneum. Typical humectants include glycerin, sorbitol, urea, alpha-hydroxy acids, and sugars.[10] Important point to remember here is that unless relative humidity is high, humectants can make skin feel tight and dry, and hence may better avoided in Mongoloid skin types and in regions of India which are semiarid and dry and in dry winter months.
- *Occlusives* physically block TEWL. Lanolin, petrolatum, silicone, zinc oxide and mineral oils are chief components.[10,11] Since lanolin is a known contact allergen, it is better to be avoided in skin types easily predisposed to contact dermatitis.[8] They may be more suitable in dry, arid conditions.
- *Emollients* contain substances like squalene, cholesterol, fatty acids and hyaluronic acid. These substances cause soothing effect to skin and may be used in individuals prone to skin hyper-reactivity.[12]
- *Natural moisturizing factor* contains low- and high-molecular weight proteins and peptides which are predominantly derived from filaggrin and

its products.[13] These are used for patients who have xerosis, atopic dermatitis and sensitive skin.

CONCLUSION

Moisturizers are integral to a dermatologist's armamentarium. However, a lot depends upon their wise selection and for that a deeper look into a patient's life may be needed while considering factors inherent to his skin and its genetics. India is a land of diversity, therefore, keeping our mind-set open with prudent observation into macro- and microenvironment of our patient's skin may be helpful in choosing a right moisturizer.

REFERENCES

1. Taylor SC. Skin of color: biology, structure, function, and implications for dermatologic disease. J Am Acad Dermatol. 2002;46(2 Suppl Understanding):S41-62.
2. Elsner P (Ed). Bioengineering of the Skin: Skin Biomechanics (Volume 5). Boca Raton, FL: CRC Press; 2002. pp. 296.
3. Kompaore F, Tsuruta H. In vivo differences between Asian, black and white in the stratum corneum barrier function. Int Arch Occup Environ Health. 1993;65(1 Suppl):S223-5.
4. Kompaore F, Marty JP, Dupont C. In vivo evaluation of the stratum corneum barrier function in blacks, Caucasians and Asians with two noninvasive methods. Skin Pharmacol. 1993;6(3):200-7.
5. Sugino K, Imokawa G, Maibach HI. Ethnic difference of stratum corneum lipid in relation to stratum corneum function. J Invest Dermatol. 1993;100(4):587.
6. Berardesca E, Elsner P, Wilhelm KP, Maibach HI (Eds). Bioengineering of the Skin: Methods and Instrumentation, 1st edition. Boca Raton, FL: CRC Press, Inc.; 1995.
7. Berardesca E, Maibach H. Cutaneous reactive hyperaemia: racial differences induced by corticoid application. Br J Dermatol. 1989;120(6):787-94.
8. Zirwas MJ, Stechschulte SA. Moisturizer allergy: diagnosis and management. J Clin Aesthet Dermatol. 2008;1(4):38-44.
9. Sagiv AE, Dikstein S, Ingber A. The efficiency of humectants as skin moisturizers in the presence of oil. Skin Res Technol. 2001;7(1):32-5.
10. Draelos ZD. Active agents in common skin care products. Plastv Reconstr Surg. 2010;125(2):719-24.
11. Ghadially R, Halkier-Sorensen L, Elias PM. Effects of petrolatum on stratum corneum structure and function. J Am Acad Dermatol. 1992;26(3):387-96.
12. Wan DC, Wong VW, Longaker MT, Yang GP, Wei FC. Moisturizing different racial skin types. J Clin Aesthet Dermatol. 2014;7(6):25-32.
13. Bolliger A, Gross R. Water soluble compounds (non-keratins) associated with the skin flakes of the human scalp. Aust J Exp Biol Med Sci. 1956;34(3):219-24.

CHAPTER 15

Natural Emollients

Narendra Gokhale

INTRODUCTION

Vegetable oils have been used since millennia for moisturizing and smoothening the skin across civilizations around the globe. Before the advent of the factory-made moisturizers, these were the only products for the said purpose. Vegetable oils as stand-alone products have fallen out of favor probably because they are messy and economical products are not marketed vociferously in the world of high decibel multimedia marketing (Table 1). On the other hand, many cosmetic companies incorporate a small amount of the exotic oils into their products so that they can shoot up the cost of the product. But they continue to form important ingredients of most of the moisturizers sold in the market today. In this chapter, we shall be looking briefly at the science behind these products.

CUTANEOUS LIPIDS AND BARRIER FUNCTION OF THE STRATUM CORNEUM

The stratum corneum is the final frontier of the skin which protects the skin from environmental damage and prevents evaporation of water from the skin. It consists of fully differentiated, anuclear, flat keratinocytes rich in keratin surrounded by a lipid matrix. The lipid matrix consists of cholesterol, ceramides, free fatty acids, and small amounts of squalene and phospholipids.

This biphasic arrangement is crucial to the barrier function of the horny layer. Any metabolic deficiencies or environmental damage which disrupts this arrangement leads to an impaired barrier function. Here in lies the role of vegetable oils rich in triglycerides and fatty acids which are taken up easily by the lipid compartment and help to restore it. Especially useful are ω6 fatty acids which are directly incorporated in the lipid layer after topical application, and hence they reduce dryness, irritation and improve the barrier function.[1] Polar triglycerides can bind to proteins reducing the binding of surfactants, and thus minimizing surfactant-induced irritation.[2]

Table 1: Vegetable oils commonly used in cosmetics

Type of oil	Constituents	Functions
Corn oil	Linoleic acid, oleic acid, palmitic acid, linolenic acid	Emulsion and moisturizer in emulsions, as a vehicle to dissolve liposoluble active ingredients like retinol
Cocoa butter	Oleic, palmitic and stearic acids	
Coconut oil/cocoa butter	95% saturated fat, lauric, myristic, caprylic, capric, palmitic acids	Sebum reconstitution properties
Palm kernel oil	Lauric, myristic, oleic and palmitic acids	Similar to coconut oil
Palm oil	Oleic and palmitic acids	Bulk quantities
Soybean oil	Oleic, linoleic, palmitic, stearic and linolenic acid. Tocopherol, phytosterols	Highly susceptible to oxidation
Rapeseed oil oxidation	Oleic, linoleic and linolenic acids, tocopherol, phytosterol	Same as soybean oil
Sunflower seed oil	Linoleic acid, tocopherols glyceryl trioleate a polar lipid	Emollient, repair process
Olive oil	Oleic 70–80%, linoleic, palmitoleic, palmitic and stearic acids, squalene	Sebum restitutive, emollient, repair process stimulation
Sweet almond oil		
Avocado oil	Oleic, linoleic, palmitic, palmitoleic acids, branched chain hydrocarbons, phytosterols, terpene alcohol, avocatine, vitamin E	Stimulates fibroblasts, inhibits collagenase used in antiaging
Borage oil	Linoleic, oleic, R-linolenic, palmitic and stearic acids	Antioxidant
Evening primrose oil	Linolenic acid, linoleic acid, polyphenols	Antioxidant
Shea butter	Oleic, stearic, linoleic, palmitic, linolenic and arachidic acids. Triterpene alcohols, cinnamates, tocopherols	

CONTENTS OF VEGETABLE OILS

Plants produce vegetable oils as a storehouse of energy, to be used when required especially in time of growth, and also to form a protective layer. The highest amounts are found in seeds, smaller quantities in pericarp of some fruits and very little in pollens, spores and vegetative organs.

Plant lipids are composed mainly of aliphatic carboxylic acids with even number of carbon atoms. Ninety-five percent of the vegetable oils are formed by a blend of triglycerides, with tiny amounts of bi- and monoglycerides. They are the primary constituents of vegetable oils. Vegetable oil triglycerides are triesters of polyol glycerin with long chain monocarboxylic fatty acids. Most fatty acids have 16 or 18 carbon atom chains. The fatty acids present naturally have *cis* configuration but the *trans* fatty acids are produced because of the oil refining process.

Coconut and palm oil contain mainly saturated fatty acids, while other oils contain mainly unsaturated fatty acids. Oleic acid, linoleic acid and linolenic acid make up almost the entire bulk of unsaturated fatty acids.

Other ingredients of the vegetable oils are called the secondary ingredients. The saponifiable fraction of the secondary ingredients includes phospholipids, glycolipids, sulfolipids, sphingolipids and waxes. The non-saponifiable fraction of vegetable oils includes, hydrocarbons like squalene, pigments in the form of carotenoids and chlorophyll, vitamin E, phytosterols, polyphenols and triterpene alcohols. These components are responsible for anti-inflammatory and antioxidant effects. Squalene peroxide is comedogenic but purification solves this problem.

Squalene is hydrogenated to produce squalane which is more stable, less oily and pleasant and light to feel.[3,4]

UNDERSTANDING TERMINOLOGIES AND BASIC CHEMISTRY RELATED TO VEGETABLE OILS

Saponifiable ingredients: The ones that can react with alkali to form soap.

Triglyceride = Glycerin + three fatty acids, no free alcohol group.

Saturated fatty acids = No double bond between carbon atoms in the acyl chain.

Unsaturated fatty acids = One or more double bonds present.

Monounsaturated fatty acid = One double bond

Polyunsaturated fatty acid = More than one double bond.

$\omega 3$, $\omega 6$ and $\omega 9$ = Among the unsaturated fatty acids, the distance of the first double bond from the first terminal methyl group in the chain categorizes them into $\omega 3$, $\omega 6$ and $\omega 9$

$\omega 9$ are monounsaturated, e.g., oleic acid; $\omega 3$, e.g., α-linolenic acid, eicosapentaenoic acid (EPA), docosahexaenoic acid (DHA) and $\omega 6$, e.g., linoleic acid, gamma linolenic acid are polyunsaturated.

Cis configuration = both chains separated by a double bond lie on the same side of the plane.

The distance of the double bond and the *cis/trans* configuration determines the biological properties.

Unsaturated fats are degraded easily on contact with air and become rancid.

The more unsaturated the molecule, lower the melting point.

Hence, products with unsaturated fats need to be mixed with antioxidants to make them stable; in contrast products with saturated fats have a long shelf life.

Oils: Triglycerides rich in unsaturated fatty acids which are liquid at room temperature.

Butters: Triglycerides rich in saturated fatty acids which are consistent and solid at room temperature. Oils can be transformed into butters by hydrogenation.

Phospholipids: Glycerin + fatty acids + phosphoric group + hydroxylated compound (choline, cholamine, serine).

Glycolipids: Glycerin + two fatty acids + galactose.

Sphingolipids: Fatty acid bound to a long-chain amino alcohol to form a ceramide.

Waxes: Complex blends of esters of long chain fatty acids with higher alcohols like docosanol, tetracosanol, and acacosanol.

Squalene, a terpene is the biosynthetic precursor of all sterols.

CLINICAL USE

Vegetable oils are excellent economical sources for maintaining the hydration of the skin[5] and to improve the barrier function where it is impaired.[6] Although traditionally, dermatologists have used mineral oil for the said purpose, vegetable oils have been found to be equally, if not more, efficacious.[7] Nanostructured lipid base formulation based on argan oil and jojoba oil with better efficacy have also been recently developed.[8]

Because of their anti-inflammatory and antimicrobial effects, vegetable oils are excellent coprescription drugs for atopic dermatitis and other eczematous disorders.[9]

OIL MASSAGE IN THE PEDIATRIC AGE GROUP

Oil massage of neonates and infants is widely practiced in India. It offers many advantages apart from moisturizing and smoothening of the skin. It helps to reduce the surfactant-induced irritation and improves the barrier function of the neonatal skin.[10] Infants undergoing massage also show better weight gain because of increased vagal activity, gastric motility, insulin-like growth factor and better thermoregulation.[11] Because of the incompletely developed barrier function of neonates, transcutaneous absorption of the oil is also more. Children massaged with safflower oil showed higher levels of serum essential fatty acids (EFAs) while those massaged with coconut oil showed more saturated fats in their blood.[12] Also it leads to a better bonding between the mother and the child.

ADVERSE EFFECTS

Considering their popularity and widespread use, the incidence of adverse effects related to vegetable oils is very low. There are isolated reports of a pityriasis-like eruption with mustard oil,[13] contact dermatitis with almond oil[14,15] and a condition called "Moodi-chud" reported from Kerala because of oil application in hot humid weather.

CONCLUSION

Vegetable oils represent economical, environment-friendly options for management of dry skin. They are a rich source of fatty acid esters that are taken up easily by the lipid component of the stratum corneum. Apart from providing good emollient effect, they also prevent transepidermal water loss and help in prevention and repair of surfactant-damaged skin. Considering their widespread use, the reported side effects are very less.

REFERENCES

1. Rigano L, Andolfatto C. Loden M, Maibach HI (Eds). Treatment of Dry Skin Syndrome. Springer; 2012. pp. 419-29.
2. Mukherjee S, Yang L, Vincent C, et al. A comparison between interactions of triglyceride oil and mineral oil with proteins and their ability to reduce cleanser surfactant induced irritation. Int J Cosmet Sci. 2015 Feb 6. doi: 10.1111/ics.12205. [Epub ahead of print].
3. Wolosik K, Knas M, Zalewska A, et al. The importance and perspective of plant-based squalene in cosmetology. J Cosmet Sci. 2013;64(1):59-66.
4. Huang ZR, Lin YK, Fang JY. Biological and pharmacological activities of squalene and related compounds: potential uses in cosmetic dermatology. Molecules. 2009;14(1):540-54.
5. Evangelista MT, Abad-Casintahan F, Lopez-Villafuerte L. The effect of topical virgin coconut oil on SCORAD index, transepidermal water loss, and skin capacitance in mild to moderate pediatric atopic dermatitis: a randomized, double-blind, clinical trial. Int J Dermatol. 2014;53(1):100-8.
6. Danby SG, AlEnezi T, Sultan A, et al. Effect of olive and sunflower seed oil on the adult skin barrier: implications for neonatal skin care. Pediatr Dermatol. 2013;30(1):42-50.
7. Agero AL, Verallo-Rowell VM. A randomized double-blind controlled trial comparing extra virgin coconut oil with mineral oil as a moisturizer for mild to moderate xerosis. Dermatitis. 2004;15(3):109-16.
8. Estanqueiro M, Conceição J, Amaral MH, et al. Characterization, sensorial evaluation and moisturizing efficacy of nanolipidgel formulations. Int J Cosmet Sci. 2014;36(2):159-66.
9. Verallo-Rowell VM, Dillague KM, Syah-Tjundawan BS. Novel antibacterial and emollient effects of coconut and virgin olive oils in adult atopic dermatitis. Dermatitis. 2008;19(6):308-15.
10. Dhar S, Banerjee R, Malakar R. Oil massage in babies: Indian perspectives. Indian J Paediatr Dermatol. 2013;14:1-3.
11. Sankaranarayanan K, Mondkar JA, Chauhan MM, et al. Oil massage in neonates: An open randomized controlled study of coconut versus mineral oil. Indian Pediatr. 2005;42(9):877-84.
12. Solanki K, Matnani M, Kale M, et al. Transcutaneous absorption of topically massaged oil in neonates. Indian Pediatr. 2005;42(10):998-1005.
13. Zawar V. Pityriasis rosea-like eruptions due to mustard oil application. Indian J Dermatol Venereol Leprol. 2005;71(4):282-4.
14. Guillet G, Guillet MH. [Percutaneous sensitization to almond oil in infancy and study of ointments in 27 children with food allergy]. Allerg Immunol (Paris). 2000;32(8):309-11.
15. Sarkar R, Basu S, Agrawal RK, et al. Skin care of the newborn. Indian Pediatr. 2010;47(7):593-8.

CHAPTER 16

Use of Moisturizers in Conditions of Hyperpigmentation

Seemal R Desai, Abhijeet K Jha, Rashmi Sarkar

INTRODUCTION

Facial hyperpigmentation and hypermelanoses are common, frustrating skin conditions that dermatologists often treat on a daily basis. These conditions can be particularly challenging to treat in patients with skin of color, and particularly those of Asian background. Though there are a variety of facial hypermelanoses, melasma and postinflammatory hyperpigmentation (PIH) are two of the most common conditions that are diagnosed and managed in the dermatologic setting.

MELASMA

Melasma is one of the most common pigmentary disorders. It is characterized by light to dark brown macules and coalescing patches that most commonly occur on the face. It is important to note that melasma can be extrafacial, and present on sites such as the upper extremities and trunk. Facial melasma can be further classified based on morphological pattern, to include centrofacial type, malar type and mandibular type.

Melasma can be a particularly challenging and difficult condition to treat. Often times, multiple treatment modalities, and extensive patient education are needed to achieve optimal results. Even then, many cases of melasma are resistant to treatment, and often times many cases do relapse. Most commonly, the relapses tend to occur due to repeat ultraviolet (UV) exposure, which is a common inciting factor in the pathogenesis of the disease. Though the severity of melasma can vary from patient to patient, it is crucial that we as dermatologists take time to educate our patients, and attempt to best elucidate the underlying cause of the patient's hyperpigmentation.

POSTINFLAMMATORY HYPERPIGMENTATION

Postinflammatory hyperpigmentation results in acquired increased melanin pigment following any skin inflammation or injury. In many patients with skin of color, one of the most common causes of PIH is acne vulgaris.

Various agents have been used to treat melasma which include hydroquinone, topical steroids, retinoic acid, and kojic acid to name a few. Chemical peels are also commonly used in treating the condition, and include glycolic acid, trichloroacetic acid, salicylic acid, lactic acid and even laser therapy from which studies have demonstrated varied success. These agents have few localized side effects such as irritation, dryness and erythema. Topical therapy remains a mainstay of treatment for melasma. Triple combination creams (modified Kligman regime) is the most commonly used topical agent for treating melasma. This therapy can have cutaneous side effects which include irritation, xerosis and erythema, which at times can be troublesome to the patient, and hence can affect patient compliance. The judicious and proper use of moisturizers in the setting of topical therapy and physical therapy for melasma can be very helpful as they are able to alleviate irritation and dryness.

MOISTURIZERS

Moisturizers simply attempt to retard transepidermal water loss and create an optimal environment for restoration of the stratum corneum barrier.[1] Occlusive moisturizers prevent evaporative water loss to the environment by placing an oily substance on the skin surface through which water cannot penetrate.[2] On the other hand, humectants attract water, similar to the functioning of dermal glycosaminoglycans. Humectants may make the skin feel smoother. Emollients make the skin smoother by repairing the skin barrier. Over the past several years, newer technologies, along with increasing demands from consumers for higher quality evidence-based products, have led to dynamic growth and changes in the antiaging skin care market. This is particularly true in the segment of skin moisturizers.

Skin moisturizers can contain a variety of different ingredients. These can include ceramides, lipid extracts, antioxidants, proteases, and even herbal extracts. *Ginkgo biloba*, green tea, aloe vera, allantoin, and licochalcone are botanical anti-inflammatory agents that are available in the current market.[3] Aloe vera and witch hazel, which were found commonly, also have skin-soothing properties.[3] Aloe vera contains 75 potentially active constituents: vitamins, enzymes, minerals, sugars, lignin, saponins, salicylic acids and amino acids.[4-6]

Aloe Vera

Aloe vera gel has been reported to have a protective effect against radiation damage to the skin.[7,8] The anti-inflammatory effect of aloe vera results from inhibition of cyclo-oxygenase pathway. Mucopolysaccharides help in binding moisture into the skin. Aloe stimulates fibroblast which produces the collagen and elastin fibers making the skin more elastic and less wrinkled. It also has cohesive effects on the superficial flaking of epidermal cells by sticking them together, which softens the skin.[9] There is no clear evidence behind use of aloe vera in melasma as a moisturizer to combat the localized adverse effects of various topical agents used to treat the condition. However, it can be potentially useful in helping to reduce the xerosis, irritation and discomfort that can be associated.

Niacinamide

Niacinamide is an active form of vitamin B3. Niacinamide is an anti-inflammatory agent and acts through inhibition of transfer of melanosomes from the melanocyte to the keratinocyte.[10,11] The cutaneous bioavailability of niacinamide is independent of the vehicle, showing good penetration and a maximum absorption rate at 48–72 hours.[12] In other hypermelanoses, such as melasma, a 4% formulation of niacinamide was able to reduce the epidermal melanin content and associated dermal inflammation, thereby improving the clinical hyperpigmentation.[13]

Vitamin C

Vitamin C is a naturally occurring antioxidant that interacts with copper ions at the tyrosinase active site. Vitamin C also acts as a reducing agent at different oxidative steps of melanin formation, thereby inhibiting melanogenesis.[14] Studies have shown that the reduced tyrosinase activity mediated by vitamin C seems to be caused by antioxidant activity, and not by the direct inhibition of tyrosinase activity.[15] Vitamin C is a constituent of many cosmeceutical products.

Boswellic Acids

Boswellic acids (BAs) are pentacyclic triterpenes, with strong anti-inflammatory activity, extracted from the gum resins of the tropical tree *Boswellia serrata*. In numerous clinical trials, specifically both *in vitro* and *in vivo* studies, BAs were found to exert significant anti-inflammatory and pro-apoptotic activity.[16] Although the mechanism of action in hyperpigmentation is not clear, it is used in many cosmetic products, and does have potential to be helpful with associated inflammation that can be seen in melasma patients.

The use of moisturizers in patients with PIH following acne sequela can be challenging at times. PIH seems to be one of the most common sequela following acne. The judicious use of non-comedogenic moisturizers can be very useful, especially given the fact that many topical acne medications can induce xerosis, irritant contact dermatitis, and even erythema. Dimethicone and glycerin are two of the most common ingredients found in various moisturizing products. Dimethicone and cyclomethicone are silicone derivatives and usually used in oil-free facial moisturizers.[17] Occlusive agents, such as petrolatum, lanolin, mineral oil, paraffin, squalene, and silicone derivatives (dimethicone, cyclomethicone) are usually greasy.[17] It is important to ensure that patients are given extensive counseling on the acne, and possible subsequent induction of PIH, from many occlusive facial agents. Silicone derivatives when combined with petrolatum, make them greasy, but if used alone seems to be non greasy. Moisturizers can have more than one ingredient, for example dimethicone, having both occlusive and emollient properties. At times various botanical and acne anti-inflammatory agents are incorporated in moisturizers for achieving a non-comedogenic property.

CONCLUSION

Although there is no evidence-based trial of using moisturizers along with other agents, the addition of various ingredients seems to be logical and also helps in improving patient's compliance.

The most important mantra in the treatment of patients with melasma, PIH, and other forms of facial hypermelanoses, is to convey that these are chronic conditions, and often involve a multimodality approach to therapy. Many topical and physical modalities can have irritating and burdensome side effects. Moisturizers and proper skin care can help to reduce those side effects if used correctly, in the patient with the correct skin type, along with sun protection, and applied consistently. This then in turn can lead to potential better patient compliance, satisfaction, and thus treatment outcomes for these patients.

REFERENCES

1. Lynde CW. Moisturizers: what they are and how they work. Skin Therapy Lett. 2001;6(13):3-5.
2. Wilhelm KP, Cua AB, Maibach HI. Skin aging. Effect on transepidermal water loss, stratum corneum hydration, skin surface pH, and casual sebum content. Arch Dermatol. 1991;127(12):1806-9.
3. Draelos ZD. Cosmetics and Dermatological Problems and Solutions, 3rd edition. London: Informa Healthcare; 2011.
4. Atherton P. Aloe vera revisited. Br J Phytother. 1998;4:76-83.
5. Shelton RM. Aloe vera. Its chemical and therapeutic properties. Int J Dermatol. 1991;30(10):679-83.
6. Atherton P. The Essential Aloe Vera: The Actions and the Evidence, 2nd edition. 1997.
7. Roberts DB, Travis EL. Acemannan-containing wound dressing gel reduces radiation-induced skin reactions in C3H mice. Int J Radiat Oncol Biol Phys. 1995;32(4):1047-52.
8. Sato Y, Ohta S, Shinoda M. [Studies on chemical protectors against radiation XXXI: Protective effects of Aloe arborescens on skin injury induced by x-irradiation]. Yakugaku Zasshi. 1990;110(11):876-84.
9. Surjushe A, Vasani R, Saple DG. Aloe vera: a short review. Indian J Dermatol. 2008;53(4):163-6.
10. Hakozaki T, Minwalla L, Zhuang J, et al. The effect of niacinamide on reducing cutaneous pigmentation and suppression of melanosome transfer. Br J Dermatol. 2002;147(1):20-31.
11. Bissett DL, Miyamoto K, Sun P, et al. Topical niacinamide produces yellowing, wrinkling, red blotchiness, and hyperpigmented spots in aging facial skin. Int J Cosmet Sci. 2004;26(5):231-8.
12. Cosmetic Ingredient Review Expert Panel. Final report of the safety assessment of niacinamide and niacin. Int J Toxicol. 2005;24 Suppl 5:1-31.
13. Navarrete-Solís J, Castanedo-Cázares JP, Torres-Álvarez B, et al. A Double-Blind, Randomized Clinical Trial of Niacinamide 4% versus Hydroquinone 4% in the Treatment of Melasma. Dermatol Res Pract. 2011;2011:379173.
14. Sarkar R, Arora P, Garg KV. Cosmeceuticals for Hyperpigmentation: What is Available? J Cutan Aesthet Surg. 2013;6(1):4-11.
15. Choi YK, Rho YK, Yoo KH, et al. Effects of vitamin C vs. multivitamin on melanogenesis: comparative study in vitro and in vivo. Int J Dermatol. 2010;49(2):218-26.
16. Moussaieff A, Mechoulam R. Boswellia resin: from religious ceremonies to medical uses; a review of in vitro, in vivo and clinical trials. J Pharm Pharmacol. 2009;61(10):1281-93.
17. Del Rosso JQ. Moisturizers: Function, formulation and clinical applications. In: Draelos Z, Dover JS, Alam M (Eds). Cosmeceuticals, 2nd edition. China: Saunders Elsevier; 2009. pp. 97-102.

CHAPTER 17

Adverse Effects of Moisturizers

Priyanka Borde Bisht, Shilpa Garg

INTRODUCTION

Moisturizers are considered very safe, especially when compared to some drugs, e.g., topical corticosteroids. However, adverse skin reactions from topical moisturizer preparations are not uncommon. Virtually any topical substance can irritate the skin, but some individuals are more susceptible than others. Atopics are particularly at risk for adverse skin reactions, due to their impaired barrier function. Facial skin is also more prone to adverse skin reactions than other body regions, possibly because of a less efficient barrier, with a smaller number of stratum corneum cell layers and the presence of large follicular pores.[1] Neonates and infants may also be prone to side effects with moisturizers.

ADVERSE EFFECTS OF MOISTURIZERS

Adverse effects which are reported with the use of moisturizers are as follows:
- *Sensory or subjective sensation*: The most common adverse reaction is the sensory or subjective sensation which is felt immediately after application of a moisturizing product. Smarting, burning and stinging sensation commonly occurs without any signs of inflammation. Preservatives, like benzoic acid and sorbic acid, and humectants, such as lactic acid, urea, pyrrolidone carboxylic acid, and sodium chloride, are well known to cause uncomfortable subjective sensations.[2] Facial skin and excoriated skin in general are most sensitive to stinging. Combinations containing corticosteroids do not eliminate this stinging. In fact, 12–30% of eczema patients using hydrocortisone creams with 4–20% urea reported stinging.[3] When atopics were asked to judge the degree of adverse skin reactions to urea-containing moisturizers, 20–40% reported smarting sensations (a sharp, local, superficial effect similar to the reaction noted to acidic solutions).[4] Some patients develop "status cosmeticus" in which every product applied to the face produces itching, burning, or stinging sensations. The use of mild soaps and shower/bath oils containing noxious substances may also constitute a risk for adverse reactions. Barrier-deteriorating substances from "mild" soaps and shower oils remain on the skin after rinsing. Repeated barrier insults with subclinical skin damage will make the skin vulnerable to further irritation and may lead to epidermal hyperplasia and inflammation.

- *Irritant and allergic dermatitis*: Moisturizers are usually free from strong irritants, however repeated application of mildly irritating preparations to sensitive areas may increase transepidermal water loss (TEWL) and cause dermatitis. Frequent immersion of the skin in water paradoxically is counterproductive to moisturization. Classic hydrophilic ointment is stabilized with emulsifying wax containing the well-known irritant sodium lauryl sulfate at a concentration of 10% as coemulsifier.[5] Aqueous solutions of 1% sodium lauryl sulfate are commonly used in experimental dermatology to induce irritation. Also fatty acids, sometimes found in moisturizers as emulsifiers, can influence skin barrier properties. Non-ionic emulsifiers, because of their mildness, are the preferred stabilizers for emulsions, but TEWL measurements indicate that some of them may also produce invisible barrier damage when applied to normal skin. Non-ionic polyethylene glycol emulsifiers are also susceptible to oxidation, inducing formation of peroxides and aldehydes. Propylene glycol may also cause adverse reactions in normal subjects at concentrations as low as 10% under occlusive conditions and in dermatitis patients at concentrations as low as 2%. The nature of the skin response has been classified into four mechanisms:
  - Subjective or sensory irritation
  - Allergic contact dermatitis
  - Non-immunologic contact urticaria
  - Irritant contact dermatitis.

Fragrances are the most frequent sensitizers in topically applied products. They have no pharmacological role, but their inclusion into creams and lotions may enhance patient compliance. The prevalence of sensitization to fragrances in eczema patients treated by dermatologists is between 6 and 14%. More than 2,000 substances are used in fragrances and over 100 have been identified as allergens.[6]

Zirwas and Stechschulte published a study utilizing database of all moisturizers available at Walgreens Pharmacy (Chicago, Illinois), which listed each product's allergens from the North American Contact Dermatitis Group (NACDG) screening panel. Of the 276 moisturizers studied, 187 (68%) contained fragrance, making it the most common allergen found in these moisturizers (Table 1). Of the products that did not contain fragrance, 43 (16%) contained fragrance-related potential allergens like benzyl alcohol or essential oils and biologic additives. Therefore, only 46 (17%) were absolutely fragrance free and definitely safe for individuals with fragrance allergy, while 230 (83%) of 276 moisturizers contained at least one ingredient to which a fragrance-allergic patient could react. The second most common allergens were parabens, commonly used as preservatives, found in 170 (62%) of the 276 products. Vitamin E, the third most common allergen found in 151 (55%) of the 276 moisturizers, is commonly added for its potential antioxidant properties. Essential oils and biologic additives, added for their fragrance, were the fourth most common allergens and were found in 123 (45%) of 276 products. Benzyl alcohol, a common fragrance and preservative, was the fifth most common allergen discovered in 65 (24%) of 276 moisturizers. Propylene glycol, a humectant and preservative, was found in 56 (20%) of 276 products, making it the sixth most common allergen. Formaldehyde releasers, used as preservatives, were grouped together and were the seventh most

Table 1: Common allergens found in 276 moisturizers[7]	
Allergen	Percentage of products containing allergen
Fragrance	67.7
Parabens	61.6
Vitamin E	54.7
Essential oils and biological additives	44.6
Benzyl alcohol	23.6
Propylene glycol	20.3
Formaldehyde-releasing preservatives	19.9
Iodopropynyl butylcarbamate	16.3
Lanolin	9.8
Kathon CG	6.2

common allergens, discovered in 55 (20%) of 276 products. Iodopropynyl butylcarbamate, a preservative, was the eighth most common allergen found in 45 (16%) of 276 products. Lanolin, a component of moisturizer used to soothe the skin, was the ninth most common allergen and was identified in 27 (10%) of 276 products. Methylisothiazolinone/methylchloroisothiazolinone is another preservative and was the 10th most common allergen in moisturizers, found in 17 (6%) of 276 available products.[7]

Product labeling of moisturizers should identify the major fragrance allergens that they contain. Patch testing to individual allergens can then be performed on persons with a history of allergy to moisturizers. This would enable these patients to avoid formulations to which they might be sensitive, just as is presently done with the testing and labeling of preservatives.

Very rarely, humectants, emulsifiers, and oils cause contact allergy.[6] Vegetable oils such as peanut oil contains proteins which can elicit sensitization reactions in allergic individuals. Lanolins are sometimes proposed to be a frequent cause of contact allergy, but this is believed to be the result of inappropriate testing conditions leading to false-positive reactions. Adverse reactions to herbal extracts are rare, probably a manifestation of the trivial amounts present in the finished product. However, virtually all herbal remedies can cause allergic reactions and several can be responsible for photosensitization. For example, aloe vera, black cumin oil, chamomile, Chinese herbal mixture, olive oil, tea tree oil and *Inula helenium*, have been reported to be able to cause allergic contact dermatitis.[8]

- *Cosmetic acne and folliculitis*: Cosmetic acne and folliculitis resulting from blockage of the follicular orifices are frequently encountered side effects of moisturizers, especially in teenagers. Application of the product in the direction of hair growth is sometimes recommended to prevent folliculitis.
- *Sweat dermatitis or miliaria*: Thick formulations can obstruct sweat gland orifices in hot, humid weather and cause sweat dermatitis or miliaria.
- *Photosensitivity or photocontact dermatitis*: This is another rare adverse effect that can be caused by wide variety of ingredients. Sunscreens, fragrances and halogenated preservatives are the most frequent offenders.
- *Systemic side effects*: Systemic side effects of moisturizers are extremely rare. Ingredients reported to be capable of inducing systemic toxicity are salicylic

acid and propylene glycol. However, intoxication has occurred. For example, topical treatment with salicylic acid in children with lamellar ichthyosis and treatment with high concentrations of propylene glycol in burn patients have resulted in poisoning.[9] When used as a preservative in cosmetics, a maximum concentration of 0.5% of salicylic acid is allowed in Europe. The acid is readily absorbed by the skin, and symptoms of salicylate poisoning have been reported after excessive application of high concentrations (>5%) to large areas of the body. Propylene glycol has been given an acceptable daily intake value of 25 mg/kg by the joint Food and Agriculture Organization/World Health Organization Expert Committee of Food. Poisoning has been found after oral doses of about 100–200 mg/kg in children and after topical treatment with high concentrations in burn patients.[10] Hence, repeated applications of high concentrations (>20%) of propylene glycol should be avoided on large body areas in children with diseased skin. Strictly certified purification of tallow from animals eliminates any risk associated with the bovine spongiform encephalopathy.
- Moreover, some products, particularly Chinese herbal creams have been shown repeatedly to be adulterated with corticosteroids, which may cause all the side effects associated with prolonged use of topical corticosteroids.

CONCLUSION

Moisturizers are considered very safe by both physicians and patients and side effects are rarely seen. They are routinely prescribed by physicians for daily care of the skin and as therapeutic moisturizers for certain dermatological conditions as well as used by people on their own. However, physicians should be aware of the side effects which can be seen due to application of moisturizers and be especially vigilant in atopic patients and in patients with known history of allergy to components of moisturizers. Hence, product labeling should be checked thoroughly by the dermatologist before prescribing any moisturizer, especially in sensitive patients.

REFERENCES

1. Berne B, Lundin Å, Malmros PE. Side effects of cosmetics and toiletries in relation to use. A retrospective study in a Swedish population. Eur J Dermatol. 1994;4:189-93.
2. Rietschel RL, Fowler JF Jr. (Eds). Fisher's Contact Dermatitis, 4th edition. Baltimore: Williams & Wilkins; 1995.
3. Khan SA. Treatment of non-inflammatory dermatoses. A double-blind comparison of 1% hydrocortisone plus 10% urea and 0.05% flucinonide. Practitioner. 1978;221(1322):265-7.
4. Lodén M, Andersson A-C, Lindberg M. The effect of two urea containing creams on dry, eczematous skin in atopic patients. II. Adverse effects. J Dermatolog Treat. 1999;10:171-5.
5. Reynolds JEF (Ed). Martindale, The Extra Pharmacopoeia, 30th edition. London: The Pharmaceutical Press; 1993.
6. De Groot AC. Sensitizing substances. In: Loden M, Maibach HI (Eds). Dry Skin and Moisturizers: Chemistry and Function. Boca Raton, FL: CRC Press; 2000. pp. 403-11.
7. Zirwas M, Stechschulte S. Moisturizer allergy diagnosis and management. J Clin Aesthet Dermatol. 2008;1(4):38-44.
8. Ernst E. Adverse effects of herbal drugs in dermatology. Br J Dermatol. 2000;143(5):923-9.
9. Drugs AAoP-Co. 'Inactive' ingredients in pharmaceutical products: update (subject review). Pediatrics. 1997;99:268-78.
10. BIBRA. Toxicity profile—Propylene glycol. Surrey, UK: BIBRA International Ltd; 1996.

CHAPTER 18

Moisturizers for Hair and Nails

Soumya Jagadeesan

INTRODUCTION

Well-groomed and lustrous hair and nails are a sign of health and beauty. Moisturizing the hair and nails help to keep them in good health. For centuries, people have used various kinds of vegetable oils for this purpose, now the cosmetic industry has caught on using moisturizers in a variety of hair and nail care products. In the present scenario, the dermatologist is expected to have a clear understanding of the various ingredients of these products, their effects and adverse effects and guide the patients regarding their judicious use. To this aim, this chapter deals with the physiology of hydration of hair and nails, the various types of moisturizers available and the situations where to use them and avoid them, so as to effectively deal with the queries and concerns of the patients.

PHYSIOLOGY OF HYDRATION OF HAIR

Chemically, around 80% of human hair is formed by the protein keratin, which has a high sulfur content. Hair is hydrophilic; it can absorb water both in its liquid and gaseous form. Hair keratins have great affinity for water and can absorb up to 40% of its own weight in water. This absorption depends on the temperature, pH and air relative humidity rate and greatly interferes with all the proprieties of the hair such as stretching ability, diameter and internal viscosity of the fibers.[1] Absorption is followed by a swelling in the hair and can result in a 10–15% increase in the hair shaft diameter and 0.5–1.0% in its length. Both absorption and swelling depends on the mean pH. Generally, an alkaline pH results in more swelling. This absorptive and swelling phenomena are of great importance in hair care products as this influences the penetration of many molecules.

Normally, the hair resists swelling beyond an extent due to the presence of bonds that preserve the reticular integrity. In certain situations like a high pH, high temperature or hair that are damaged by weathering or by chemical treatment, the cuticle will become more porous, resulting in excessive absorption of water, swelling and damage to the hair shaft. Moreover, the hair will be unable to retain the moisture thus gained and will evaporate quickly becoming more dry.[1,2]

MOISTURIZERS FOR HAIR

Dry hair is hair which does not possess adequate moisture. It becomes difficult to style such hair and the hair loses its shine. This is usually because the cuticle has become heavily weathered and porous in damaged hair, mostly as a consequence of repeated cosmetic procedures. Treatment of dry and damaged hair consists of optimal moisturization. The essential qualification of a moisturizer is the ability to improve or maintain hydration levels of hair or skin. Appropriate levels of moisture help maintain the keratin structure and mechanical integrity of the hair. Hair with optimal water levels has more body, bounce, and looks healthy and shiny.[3]

Moisturizers for hair, as in skin are mainly classified as humectants and emollients.

Humectants

Humectants are the "true" moisturizers. They are compounds that draw moisture from the atmosphere and pull it into the hairs' cortex. This happens slowly, over an extended period of time. Humectants work at a molecular level forming hydrogen bonds with the water molecules. Humectants are generally added to shampoos, bath gels and body washes at 2–5% by weight, to prevent the formation of a surface coating. They can reduce the foam volume of the product, which may adversely affect customer satisfaction. There is a general impression created that if humectants are added to a shampoo, it will moisturize the hair shaft. Unless the molecule used is a large polymer and hygroscopic, it is not certain how much of it will be left after rinsing and washing the shampoo. This is different from a leave-on conditioner, where the humectants stays on as a thin film till it is washed off.[4]

Moreover, weather is an important factor to consider when we choose the type of product to use on the hair. In dry or low humid conditions, there isn't a lot of water in the air for the hair to draw moisture from. In this scenario, as per the laws of diffusion, there is a probability that humectants may remove the moisture from the hair cortex into the air, resulting in dry and frizzy hair. On the other hand, in wet and extremely humid conditions, if a product high in humectants, especially glycerin is used, the hair can absorb a lot of moisture from the air, causing swelling of the hair shaft, as discussed above, and damage to the cuticle, resulting in dry and sticky hair. Therefore, humectants are good in middle dew points and should be used with caution in extreme weathers.

Few examples of the humectants that are commonly used on hair are: glycerin, propylene glycol, agave nectar, fructose, sodium pyrrolidone carboxylic acid (PCA), honey, sorbitol, panthenol, hydrolyzed silk protein, etc.

Emollients

Emollients also known as sealants or antihumectants are not "true" moisturizers of the hair even though the terms are often used interchangeably. They do not actually supply moisture to the hair but rather form films/coating on the surface of the hair which seals the cuticle and traps the moisture inside. They are lubricants and provide increased slip between adjacent hair strands, which helps in detangling and smoothens and flattens the cuticle surface. They enhance the shine, softness and the flexibility of the hair fibers.

Common emollients include silicones (dimethicone, amodimethicone, cyclomethicone, etc.), fatty alcohols, petrolatum, fruit and vegetable-derived oils and butters, mineral oils, proteins, hydrolyzed proteins and polyquaterniums (cationic polymers). The selection of the appropriate emollient is important for enhancing the health and appearance of the hair strands.[5]

Many of the emollients mentioned above are entirely hydrophobic, but hydrolyzed proteins and fruit and vegetable oils are smaller molecules with fatty acid components that are hydrophilic. This property enables these to act as both emollients and as mild humectants. They can also penetrate through the cuticle layer into the cortex and significantly improve the mechanical properties of the hair. For example, coconut oil and jojoba oil are light molecules which can act as humectants as well, and coconut oil in addition can enter the hair. The selection of the emollient also depends on the hair type. Fine strands can easily clump together and can be weighed down by some oils, whereas coarser hair require heavier oils and butters. The timing of the application is also important. The hair has to be sealed with the agent after moisturization. If the emollient is applied before moisturization in very dry hair, it can prevent absorption of moisture into the hair and can cause more damage.

Hair Conditioners

A hair conditioner is an agent which when applied on the hair, improves the surface properties of the hair. Conditioners protect the edges of the cuticle scales, although they cannot repair any damage to the cortex if it has occurred. They generally contain large molecules that collect on the edges of the damaged scales of the cuticle, helping to smooth over and repair the fractures and fissures. Moisturizing agents are one of the most important ingredients of any conditioner, though they contain many other ingredients as well. Cationic polymers, hydrolyzed proteins, and silicones, such as dimethicone, are the usually seen ingredients in a conditioner, and are useful in repairing dry and damaged hair. In addition, panthenol is absorbed into the shaft and acts as a humectant by providing moisture. Dedicated products may also provide sun protection and minimize thermal damage. Some may improve color retention and add volume as well. The benefits provided by some of them may be temporary which requires frequent reapplication while others provide long-term benefit and repair damage on a daily basis.

Two-in-one Shampoos

Silicones are mainly used in 2-in-1 conditioning shampoos. Dimethicone is the silicone preferred in most products as it gives a good performance in shampoo formulations, without causing excessive build-up. In excessively damaged hair, cationic polymers are sometimes used. The conditioning from 2-in-1 conditioning shampoos is expected to occur at the rinsing stage, when the shampoo emulsion breaks and the silicone is free to deposit on the hair. The separation of cleaning and conditioning stages allow for both the functions to be performed efficiently. However, the conditioning by 2-in-1 shampoos was found to be inferior to that performed by stand-alone conditioners, and the silicones may reduce foam volume, lowering customer satisfaction with a shampoo product.[6]

Moisturization of hair can be summarized into the following:
- An effective moisturizer must contain water, emollients and humectants
- The selection of the appropriate product has to be always individualized depending on the hair characteristics, previous chemical damage, weather conditions, etc.
- Humectant-rich products should not be overused in extremely dry or wet weathers
- Emollients should be applied after moisturization of hair, to prevent leakage of moisture
- Most conditioners contain moisturizers besides other ingredients. They help repair damage that has occurred in the cuticles and improve the surface properties of the hair.

MOISTURIZERS FOR NAILS

Physiology of Hydration of Nails

The nail is a keratinized tissue, which is rich in hard keratins that have high content of cysteine, a sulfur containing amino acid. 10% of the dry weight of nail is formed by sulfur and the sulfur containing keratins are responsible for the toughness of the nail and also the excellent barrier function (making it impermeable to many substances). Lipid content of the nails is low, 0.1–1%, when compared to the 10% in stratum corneum. Water concentration is also low, 7–12%, as against 15–25% in the stratum corneum. But the nail is highly permeable to water; when its water content increases the nail becomes soft and opaque, and when the water level comes down, the nail becomes dry and brittle.

The permeability of nail is an important issue, especially when it concerns the penetration of topical medications and cosmetic agents. As a barrier, studies have shown that the nail plate reacts like a hydrogel, as opposed to the epidermis, which is a lipophilic membrane.[7]

Brittle Nails

Brittle nails are the equivalent of dry skin. Water is the plasticizer for both skin and nails. Water allows for the nails to bend without cracking. Once the water is lost, it is not possible to permanently replace it. The best treatment for brittle nails is to prevent damage to the growing nail plate. Patients must be advised to avoid frequent exposure to surfactants and solvents as they can dehydrate the nail plate. The frequent use of hand sanitizers, soaps and other household cleaning agents can be an important cause of nail damage. Soaking of nails also do not hydrate the nail, rather it promotes water loss. Acetone, present in nail polish removers can also dehydrate the nail plate, therefore its use must be minimized to protect the nail plate.

Nail Moisturizers

Urea and lactic acid are thought to promote hydration of nails by virtue of their keratolytic action. They are classified as humectants as they increase the water-holding capacity of the nails. This occurs from digestion of nail keratin that opens up water-binding sites and enhances hydration. The benefits are short lasting however and require frequent reapplication. The concentration of urea recommended is between 5 and 20% and that of lactic acid is between 5 and 10%.[8]

Other moisturizers or hydrators like glycerin, petrolatum, beeswax and a variety of mineral oils are used in hydrating the nails by sealing the moisture. Besides the nail plate, cuticle area and the skin surrounding the nails are also protected using moisturizers. Cuticle creams and conditioners generally contain common moisturizing, softening and other skin conditioning agents. Some of the most common ingredients are natural oils (almond, avocado, jojoba, and sunflower), waxes (cetyl alcohol, stearyl alcohol, and beeswax), and humectants (aloe vera, ceramides, and glycerin).

Nail Hardeners

There are two types of nail hardeners available: crosslinking hardeners and reinforcing hardeners.

Crosslinking Hardeners

They react with the protein in the nails, making it stronger. They create chemical bonds that cross-link the protein chains together to make the nails harder. Some common ingredients include formaldehyde. Though they increase hardness, they reduce flexibility and should be used with caution as their frequent and long-term use can dehydrate the nail plate and make it brittle, in a paradoxical manner. They should be applied to the free edge of the nail alone and avoided altogether if possible.

Reinforcing Hardeners

This type has ingredients that coat the nail, they add a layer on the nails to reinforce their natural structure. These products use ingredients like silicum, mandelic acid, sulfhydryl protein, etc. They need to be reapplied frequently to maintain the benefits. They are thought to make the nails harder and prevents splitting and breaking.[7]

Moisturization of nails can be summarized into the following:
- Moisturizing nails help to maintain them healthy and shining
- Patients must be advised to avoid frequent use of harsh soaps, cleansing agents, formaldehyde-containing products and acetone to prevent dehydration of the nail plate
- Frequent and liberal application of moisturizing creams and lotions containing natural oils, waxes and humectants to the nail plate, surrounding skin and cuticles is recommended to maintain hydration

- Urea and lactic acid are also found to be highly effective in hydrating the nails
- Frequent soaking in water may result in brittle nails.

CONCLUSION

The appearance of a person's hair and nails is becoming increasingly important in today's world. This influences both self-perception and the way one is viewed by others. Grooming and caring of hair has been traditionally given a lot of importance in our society, especially among women—hair has been considered a woman's richest ornament. But that has not been the case with nails. However, over the last few decades trends have changed and nail grooming and nail cosmetics have also come up in a big way. The appearance of hair and nails is now taken as an index of sophistication and style, and thus maintaining adequate hydration becomes extremely important to preserve their health and beauty. Moisturizers consequently have become an indispensable part of hair and nail care. Therefore, it has become obligatory that the dermatologists keep themselves well-versed regarding these products to address the patient needs effectively. This becomes all the more important given the scant attention given to this topic in the curriculum and the limited literature available on this subject.

REFERENCES

1. Robbins CR, Crawford RJ. Cuticle damage and the tensile properties of human hair. J Soc Cosmet Chem. 1991;42:59-67.
2. Velasco MV, Dias TC, Freitas AZ, et al. Hair fiber characteristics and methods to evaluate hair physical and mechanical properties. Braz J Pharm Sci. 2009;45;153-62.
3. Trüeb RM. Pharmacologic interventions in aging hair. Clin Interv Aging. 2006;1(2):121-9.
4. Gesslein BW. Humectants in personal care formulation: A practical guide. In: Schueller R, Romanowski P (Eds). Conditioning Agents for Hair and Skin. New York: Marcel Dekker Inc.; 1999.
5. Carson J, Gallagher KF. Emollient esters and oils. In: Schueller R, Romanowski P (Eds). Conditioning Agents for Hair and Skin. New York: Marcel Dekker Inc.; 1999.
6. Kozubal C, Baca AL, Navaro E. Hair conditioners. In: Barel AO, Paye M, Maibach HI (Eds). Handbook of Cosmetic Science and Technology, 4th edition. Florida: CRC Press; 2014.
7. Andre J, Scheers C, Baran R. Normal nail and use of nail cosmetics and treatments. In: Barel AO, Paye M, Maibach HI (Eds). Handbook of Cosmetic Science and Technology, 4th edition. Florida: CRC Press; 2014.
8. Draelos ZD (Ed). Understanding and treating brittle nails. Cosmetics and Dermatologic Problems and Solutions, 3rd edition. Florida: Informa Health Care; 2011.

CHAPTER 19

Recent Update on Moisturizers

Anupam Das, Rashmi Sarkar

INTRODUCTION

The term 'moisturizer' is a generic term which encompasses numerous formulations providing therapeutically desirable effects on the skin like reduced transepidermal water loss, barrier repair, and/or esthetic improvement of skin. Softness of the skin depends on the water content. So, better the cutaneous hydration is maintained, better is the outcome.[1] Moisturizers can be divided into four classes: (1) emollients, (2) humectants, (3) occlusives, and (4) therapeutic.[2]

NEW CONCEPTS OF HYDRATION

With the advent of molecular biology and the vast developments in the field of medical sciences, we have gained a lot of knowledge regarding the hydration milieu of the skin. This has led to the development of numerous formulations with an aim to combat the deficiencies in the pathophysiology of xerosis.

- *Natural moisturizing factor*: Jacobi, in 1959 had described the role of a catabolic product of filaggrin [natural moisturizing factor (NMF)] in the maintenance of cutaneous hydration.[3-5] Natural moisturizing factor basically provides protection from skin damage by increasing the plasticity of the skin. Besides, the proper functioning of hydrolytic enzymes for desquamation requires the presence of NMF. In addition, NMF has been found to substantially contribute to the barrier function of stratum corneum. Natural moisturizing factor contains pyrrolidone carboxylic acid (PCA), urocanic acid, inorganic salts, sugars, lactic acid, and urea.[6,7] Its levels are reduced in atopic dermatitis, xerosis, psoriasis, and ichthyosis. In consistence with these facts, topical PCA has been found to improve xerosis. Besides, urea and lactate have been used since decades.[7] Moreover, urea (and its precursor arginine), has been shown to provide improvement in elderly patients with atopic dermatitis, by stimulating the expression of enzymes involved in ceramide synthesis.[8,9] Urea uptake enhances the barrier function and antimicrobial defense mechanisms in human beings by regulating epidermal gene expression.[9] L-lactic acid and D,L-lactic acid stimulate the synthesis of ceramides in the stratum corneum.[10]

- *Lipids*: Ceramides (50%), free fatty acids (15%), and cholesterol (25%) are the predominant lipid constituents of the skin.[11,12] The basic function of ceramides is reduction of water loss. Formulations containing ceramides, cholesterol, fatty acids, alpha-hydroxy radicals, humectants (glycerol and urea) have been found to provide dramatic relief to patients with xerosis.
- *Aquaporins*: Thirteen classes of this water transporter are present in mammals. However, aquaporin (AQP) 3 is the most abundant variety in the skin present in the epidermal keratinocytes. The expression is inversely proportional to age and sun exposure, thus leading to xerosis in the geriatric population. The levels are reduced in psoriatic lesions as well.[13] Substances and extracts which increase the levels of AQPs by enhancing the transcription and translation of the protein have been found to be beneficial in the treatment of xerosis. Latest ones include the herbal medicine byakkokaninjinto, an extract from the bark of *Piptadenia colubrina* (leguminous tree from South America), and an extract of *Ajuga turkestanica* (Central Asia).[14-16] Byakkokaninjinto is a herbal medicine used for the relief of diuresis, thirst, and diabetes-associated pruritus. Byakkokaninjinto treatment relieves diuresis, thirst, and dermal pruritus by increasing kidney AQP2 expression and skin AQP3 expression. Another compound, glyceryl glucoside, a chemical derivative of glycerol, has been shown to increase the levels of AQP3.[17]

NEWER MOISTURIZERS

- *Moisturizer containing sodium, potassium, and ammonium lactates* (AmLactin Lotion and Cream, Upsher-Smith Laboratories, Inc.): The formulation is well suited for rough, flaky, and dry skin. The restoring body lotion is fast-acting and long-lasting. The moisturizing body lotion gently exfoliates the skin and leads to intense hydration. The hydrating cream formulation smoothens, repairs, and softens severely dry skin. All AmLactin moisturizers contain alpha-hydroxy acids (AHAs) that are pH balanced for the skin and gently exfoliate.
- *Moisturizer containing sodium lactate and urea* (Eucerin Repair Lotions and Cream, Beiersdorf Inc.) which provide 24-hour moisture to replenish, strengthen, and protect skin.
- *Moisturizer containing arginine and sodium PCA* (Cetaphil Restoraderm, Galderma Laboratories, LP).
- *Moisturizer containing ceramides, which restore the barrier properties of the skin* (CeraVe Cream and Lotions, Valeant Pharmaceuticals North America LLC; Eucerin Smoothing Repair and Professional Repair, Beiersdorf Inc.): All CeraVe products contain the vital ceramides healthy skin needs to help restore and maintain its natural protective barrier which includes purified water, glycerin, ceteareth-20 and cetearyl alcohol, caprylic/capric triglyceride, behentrimonium methosulfate, cetearyl alcohol, cetyl alcohol, ceramide 3, ceramide 6-II, ceramide 1, hyaluronic acid, cholesterol, petrolatum, dimethicone, potassium phosphate, dipotassium phosphate, sodium lauroyl lactylate, disodium ethylenediaminetetraacetic acid, phenoxyethanol, methylparaben, propylparaben, phytosphingosine, carbomer, xanthan gum, etc.

- *Moisturizer containing synthetic derivatives of naturally occurring ceramides* (Curel Ultra Healing, Kao USA Inc.) which are formulated specifically to moisturize and heal dry skin and to prevent dry skin from recurring over time. With olive oil and fruit extracts, this preparation safely loosens flakes for superior hydration and this is clinically proven to be very beneficial for psoriasis and keratosis pilaris.
- *Moisturizer containing ceramide precursors* (hydroxypalmitoyl sphinganine) which are converted to ceramides after being applied to the skin (Cetaphil Restoraderm, Galderma Laboratories, LP).
- *Newest formulations* containing NMF, ceramide (Physiogel cream and lotion), AQP modulators, urea, lactate, arginine, and eight other amino acids. They also contain ceramide 3 and glyceryl glucoside.[18]
- *Argan oil*: It is a plant oil produced from the kernels of the *Argania spinosa* found in Morocco. The plant is well adapted to nutritionally deficient soils. It is now referred to as *Argania cosmetica*. The fruit of *A. spinosa* has an oleaginous kernel from which a well-known oil, 'argan oil', is used in folk medicine and in cosmetics.[19] It contains vitamin E, phenols, carotenes, squalene, fatty acids (80% unsaturated fatty acids),[20] caffeic acid, oleuropein, vanillic acid, tyrosol, catechol, resorcinol, (−)-epicatechin and (+)-catechin.[21,22] Over the past 15 years, cosmetic argan oil has become one of the prime focus of interest in dermocosmetology. Cosmetic argan oil is produced by solvent-assisted extraction of the finely crushed kernels. However, enriched-argan oil is produced by distillation of cosmetic argan oil, and it can be supplemented with antioxidants. Argan fruit pulp and leaves contain proteins, peptides, saponins, etc. which are highly coveted dermocosmetics these days.[23]

Traditionally, cosmetic argan oil was used in the treatment of acne, chicken pox lesions, and scars. It is also recommended to reduce xerosis and slow down the appearance of wrinkles. This oil is also used to treat joint pain, skin inflammation, psoriasis, eczema, scabies, burns, wounds, brittle fingernails, hair loss, and dry hair.[24] Cosmetic and enriched argan oils are an important component of various creams owing to their moisturizing properties. These oils have been claimed to hydrate the skin, neutralize free radicals, heal acne blemishes, reduce scars, and improve elasticity of skin.[25]

THERAPEUTIC MOISTURIZERS: CONCEPT AND BRIEF REVIEW

In an attempt to create the 'perfect' moisturizer and make it a multitasking formulation, numerous ingredients are being added to moisturizers to enhance their therapeutic potential. The various ingredients have been reviewed here.[26]
- *Sodium PCA*: It is a salt of 2-pyrrolidone-5-carboxylic acid, used in concentrations of more than 2%. It basically functions as a humectant (holds water) and acts like a 'duplicate dermis'; mimicking the dermis in its property of possessing glycosaminoglycans and holding water.[27]
- *Urea*: It has a three-fold action. Firstly, it exposes the water-holding sites of corneocytes, thus promoting moisture. Secondly, it dissolves the cementing substance and enhances desquamation. Third, it increases the water-holding capability of stratum corneum.[28]

- *Alpha-hydroxy acids (anti-aging moisturizer)*: The important ones are glycolic acid, malic acid, and citric acid. Recently, trihydroxy acids (THAs) have been launched which are prepared by combining the parent compounds. These acids lead to exfoliation of the skin leading to rejuvenation. After the application of the acids, the modified pH of stratum corneum persists for as long as 2 hours. This leads to a number of epidermal and dermal changes, the depth of change being directly proportional to the concentration of the acid.[29]
- *Beta-hydroxy acids*: Salicylic acid is the most vital member of this group and it is a well-known exfoliant. It is added to exfoliant moisturizers, preferably containing a sunscreen, and exfoliant cleansers or toners.[30]
- *Polyhydroxy acids*: These have been added to moisturizing compositions and their advantage lies in the fact that they do not produce much stinging, burning, and irritation. These are mostly used in rosacea, perioral dermatitis, and atopic dermatitis.
- *Vitamin A*: It is added to moisturizers to incorporate the 'humectant' property of retinoids. They effectively draw water from the upper dermis to epidermis.
- *Vitamin E*: Addition of this vitamin leads to improved moisturization, increased softness, and better smoothness.[31,32]
- *Panthenol*: Panthenol is enzymatically converted to pantothenic acid in skin and it is a well-known humectant vitamin. It is used as a skin-conditioning and hair-conditioning agent in shampoos, moisturizers, and hair sprays.
- *Niacinamide*: It has a unique property of water solubility and stability in the presence of light and oxygen. Researchers have found two interesting characteristics of niacinamide. It prevents photocarcinogenesis and it possesses antitumor properties; and because of these recent developments, the role of niacinamide as an efficacious moisturizer is being investigated
- *Physiological lipids*: These therapeutically resemble skin lipids like phospholipids, triglycerides, squalene, cholestrol, ceramides (Physiogel lotion and cream).

CONCLUSION

To conclude, moisturizers constitute an indispensable component of a dermatologist's prescription. They not only make the skin moist, but the addition of carefully selected components make it even more attractive to the patient and serve as a handy formulation for the prescribing clinician as well.

REFERENCES

1. Dhar S. Topical therapy of atopic dermatitis. Indian J Paediatr Dermatol. 2013;14:4-8.
2. Draelos ZD. Modern moisturizer myths, misconceptions, and truths. Cutis. 2013;91:308-14.
3. Jacobi OK. About the mechanism of moisture regulation in the horny layer of the skin. Proc Sci Sect Toilet Goods Assoc. 1959;31:22-4.
4. Fowler J. Understanding the role of natural moisturizing factor in skin hydration. Pract Dermatol. 2012:36-40.
5. Irvine AD, McLean WH, Leung DY. Filaggrin mutations associated with skin and allergic diseases. N Engl J Med. 2011;365:1315-27.
6. Weber TM, Schoelermann AM, Breitenbach U, et al. Hand and foot moisturizers. In: Draelos ZD (Ed). Cosmetic Dermatology: Products and Procedures. Hoboken, NJ: Blackwell Publishing Ltd; 2010. pp. 130-8.

7. Harding CR, Watkinson A, Rawlings AV, et al. Dry skin, moisturization and corneodesmolysis. Int J Cosmet Sci. 2000;22:21-52.
8. Lodén M. Role of topical emollients and moisturizers in the treatment of dry skin barrier disorders. Am J Clin Dermatol. 2003;4:771-88.
9. Nenoff P, Donaubauer K, Arndt T, et al. Topically applied arginine hydrochloride. Effect on urea content of stratum corneum and skin hydration in atopic eczema and skin aging [in German]. Hautarzt. 2004;55:58-64.
10. Rawlings AV, Davies A, Carlomusto M, et al. Effect of lactic acid isomers on keratinocyte ceramide synthesis, stratum corneum lipid levels and stratum corneum barrier function. Arch Dermatol Res. 1996;288:383-90.
11. Jungersted JM, Hellgren LI, Jemec GB, et al. Lipids and skin barrier function—a clinical perspective. Contact Dermatitis. 2008;58:255-62.
12. Feingold KR. Thematic review series: skin lipids. The role of epidermal lipids in cutaneous permeability barrier homeostasis. J Lipid Res. 2007;48:2531-46.
13. Lee Y, Je YJ, Lee SS, et al. Changes in transepidermal water loss and skin hydration according to expression of aquaporin-3 in psoriasis. Ann Dermatol. 2012;24:168-74.
14. Aburada T, Ikarashi N, Kagami M, et al. Byakkokaninjinto prevents body water loss by increasing the expression of kidney aquaporin-2 and skin aquaporin-3 in KKAy mice. Phytother Res. 2011;25:897-903.
15. Pereda Mdel C, Dieamant Gde C, Eberlin S, et al. Expression of differential genes involved in the maintenance of water balance in human skin by Piptadenia colubrina extract. J Cosmet Dermatol. 2010;9:35-43.
16. Dumas M, Sadick NS, Noblesse E, et al. Hydrating skin by stimulating biosynthesis of aquaporins. J Drugs Dermatol. 2007;6:s20-4.
17. Schrader A, Siefken W, Kueper T, et al. Effects of glyceryl glucoside on AQP3 expression, barrier function and hydration of human skin. Skin Pharmacol Physiol. 2012;25:192-9.
18. Weber TM, Kausch M, Rippke F, et al. Treatment of xerosis with a topical formulation containing glyceryl glucoside, natural moisturizing factors, and ceramide. J Clin Aesthet Dermatol. 2012;5:29-39.
19. Guillaume D, Charrouf Z. Argan oil and other argan products: Use in dermocosmetology. Eur J Lipid Sci Technol. 2011;113:403-8.
20. Charrouf Z, Guillaume D. Argan oil: Occurrence, composition and impact on human health. European Journal of Lipid Science and Technology. 2008;110:632.
21. Monfalouti HE, Guillaume D, Denhez C, et al. Therapeutic potential of argan oil: a review. J Pharm Pharmacol. 2010;62:1669-75.
22. Charrouf Z, Guillaume D. Phenols and Polyphenols from Argania spinosa. American Journal of Food Technology. 2007;2:679.
23. Charrouf Z, Guillaume D. Argan oil: occurrence, composition and impact on human health. The European Journal of Lipid Science and Technology. 2008;110:632-6.
24. Charrouf Z, Guillaume D. Ethnoeconomical, ethnomedical, and phytochemical study of Argania spinosa (L.) Skeels. J Ethnopharmacol. 1999;67:7-14.
25. Breton L, Jourdain R, Gueniche A, et. al. Cosmetic and/or dermatological composition for prevention and/or treatment of sensitive or dry skin US patent 2009/0232785 L'Oreal, France, 2009.
26. Draelos ZD. Therapeutic moisturizers. Dermatol Clin. 2000;18:597-607.
27. Wilkinson JB, Moore RJ. Harry's Cosmeticology, 7th edition. New York: Chemical Publishing; 1982. pp. 62-4.
28. Raab WP. Uses of urea in cosmetology. Cosmet Toilet. 1990;105:97-102.
29. Smith WP. Hydroxy acids and skin aging. Cosmet Toilet. 1994;109:41-8.
30. Draelos ZD. Hydroxy acids for the treatment of aging skin. J Geriatr Dermatol. 1997;5:236-40.
31. Idson B. Vitamins and the skin. Cosmet Toilet. 1993;108:79-92.
32. Mayer P, Pittermann W, Wallat S. The effects of vitamin E on the skin. Cosmet Toilet. 1993;108:99-109.

APPENDIX

List of Moisturizers

Name of the product	Ingredients
Dermoys cream for dry skin	- White soft paraffin IP 13.2% w/w, liquid paraffin IP 10.2% w/w - Cream base - Non-greasy - Lanolin free - Perfume free - Odor free
Parasoft cream for dry skin	- White soft paraffin IP 13.2% w/w, liquid paraffin IP 10.2% w/w Preservatives - Methyl paraben IP 0.15% w/w, propyl paraben IP 0.05% w/w in aloe vera containing cream base
Parasoft lotion	LLP, grape seed oil, avocado oil, aloe vera, jojoba oil, olive oil, BHT, BHA
Parasoft body milk	*Olea europaea* fruit oil, isoamyl laurate, *Mangifera indica* seed extract, vitamin B3, pantothenol, glycerin, *Butyrospermum parkii*, lecithin, sodium acrylate copolymer, aloe vera leaf extract
Parasoft soap	Glycerin, aloe vera, LLP, olive oil, jojoba oil, vitamin E
Parasoft baby soap	Oil, almond oil, glycerin, aloe vera, olive oil, jojoba oil, vitamin E, hydrolyzed wheat protein, shea butter
Dermadew aloe lotion	Composition: - Aloe vera gel 10% w/w, glycerin 10% w/w in a moisturizing lotion base containing dimethicone and hydrogenated polydecene Ingredients: - Purified water, octyl palmitate, dimethicone fluid, hydrogenated polydecene, cetyl alcohol, Tween-20, Olivem-800, stearic acid, perfume, pemulen TR-1, potassium sorbate, triethanolamine, methyl paraben, ultrez-10, propyl paraben
Venusia Max intense moisturizing cream	Purified water, propylene glycol, emulsifying wax, glycerin, cyclomethicone, shea butter, aloe butter, mango butter, cocoa butter, cetyl alcohol, stearic acid, dimethicone, methyl paraben, propyl paraben, disodium edentate, zinc oxide, fragrance
Atopiclair cream Relief from dry and sensitive skin, fragrance free	Aqua, ethylhexyl palmitate, *Butyrospermum parkii* butter, pentylene glycol, arachidyl alcohol, behenyl alcohol, arachidyl glucoside, butylene glycol, glyceryl stearate, PEG-100 stearate, glycyrrhetinic acid, capryloyl glycerin, bisabolol, tocopheryl acetate, carbomer, ethylhexyl glycerin, piroctone olamine, sodium hydroxide, allantoin, DMDM hydantoin, *Vitis vinifera* seed extract, sodium hyaluronate, disodium EDTA, ascorbyl tetraisopalmitate, propyl gallate, telmesteine

Continued

Continued

Name of the product	Ingredients
Dersil cream	Aloe vera extract 10% w/v, vitamin E acetate 0.5% w/v, jojoba oil 1% w/v, white soft paraffin 13.2% w/w, LLP 10.2% w/v, cream base
Glurea cream intensive repair	Urea 10% w/w, glycerin 10% w/w, cyclomethicone 1% w/w, allantoin 0.5% w/w, white petrolatum jelly 0.5% w/w, LLP, cetostearyl alcohol, stearic acid, methyl paraben, propyl paraben, ethylenediamine tetra acetate, purified water
Atogla cream	Key ingredients: • Cholesterol 0.3%, ceramide III 0.2%, oat lipid 0.2%, anti-irritant complex 0.2%, gamma linolenic acid 0.2% (from borage oil), aloe vera gel, vitamin E
Liquid paraffin heavy	Liquid Paraffin heavy
Glycerin	Glycerin
Xerina cream	Purified water (pH balanced with ammonia solution), glycolic acid, urea, cetylated fatty ester complex, ammonium hydroxide, glycerin, glyceryl monostearate, cetostearyl alcohol, PEG 100 stearate, cetyl palmitate, propylene glycol, vitamin E acetate, stearic acid, isopropyl myristate, olive oil, sepiplus, dimethicone, perfume, methyl paraben, disodium EDTA, propyl paraben
Moisturex emollient, humectant and keratolytic cream	Composition: • Urea 10% w/w, lactic acid IP 10% w/w, propylene glycol IP 10% w/w, LLP IP 10% w/w, cream base Preservatives: • Methyl paraben IP 0.16% w/w, propyl paraben IP 0.04% w/w
Acnemoist cream	Pentavitin 1% w/w, jojoba ester 3% w/w, octyl methoxycinnamate (OMC) 5%, MBBT 4%
Atogla lotion	Key ingredients: • Cholesterol 0.3%, ceramide III 0.2%, oat lipid 0.2%, anti-irritant complex 0.2%, gamma linolenic acid 0.2% (from borage oil)
Lozisoft cream and lotion	LLP 10.2%, white soft paraffin 13.2%, aloe vera 3%
Logifeel cream	Glycolic acid 15% w/w, urea 10% w/w, cetylated fatty ester complex
NMFe skin lotion	Key ingredients: • Aloe vera extract 10% w/v, vitamin E acetate 0.5% w/v in a moisturizing oil in water emulsion base Other ingredients: • Water, liquid paraffin (light), glycerin, cetostearyl alcohol, fragrance, stearic acid, cetomacrogol (1000), simethicone, methyl paraben, triethanolamine, propyl paraben, disodium edentate
Moiz moisturising cream	Cetyl alcohol IP 2% w/w in a cream base (with Silkflow-364 NF, Olivem-700, caprylic/capric triglyceride, C12-15 alkyl benzoate, Dow Corning® CB 3021)
Moiz MM, maximum moisturising cream	Cetyl alcohol IP 2% w/w, hydrogenated polydecenes, shea butter, Silkflow-366 NF, caprylic/capric triglyceride, C12-15 alkyl benzoate, glycerin, propylene glycol, LLP, stearic acid

Continued

Continued

Name of the product	Ingredients
Moiz LMF 48 lotion the long lasting moisturiser	Xylitylglucoside, anhydroxylitol, xylitol, C14-22 alcohols, C12-20 alkyl glucoside, hyaluronic acid, sodium PCA, sodium lactate, sodium gluconate, glycerin, hydroxyethyl urea, macadamia oil, phytosqualene, vitamin E, cetyl alcohol, stearyl alcohol, hydrogenated polyisobutene, caprylic/capric triglyceride
Moiz moisturising syndet bar (pH 5.5)	With syndet base, shea butter, aloe vera, vitamin E
Cetaphil moisturising cream	Polyglyceryl methacrylate, propylene glycol, glycerin, dicaprylyl ether, cetyl alcohol, sweet almond oil, dimethicone, dimethiconol, light mineral oil
Cetaphil moisturising lotion	Glycerin, hydrogenated polyisobutene, macadamia nut oil, dimethicone, stearoxytrimethylsilane, stearyl alcohol, dexpanthenol
Cetaphil DAM	Sodium PCA, panthenol, shea butter, cyclopentasiloxane, dimethiconol, ERC-5 (epidermal replenishing complex)
Efaderma	Sodium PCA 2.5%, sodium lactate 2%, sunflower oil 10%
Cetaphil daylong after sun repair lotion	Micrococcus lysate 0.005%, lecithin 0.005%, squalene 5%, shea butter 2%, panthenol 1%, tocopherol 1%, liposomal lotion
Cetaphil dermacontrol moisturizer SPF30+	Glycerin, panthenol, pentylene glycol, zinc gluconate, silica, polymethyl methacrylate, avobenzone 3%, octisalate 5%, octocrylane 5%, hydroxypalmitoyl sphinganine, allantoin, glycyrrhetinic acid, isopropyl lauryl sarcosinate, dimethicone, dimethiconol, capryl glycol
Cetaphil restoraderm moisturising lotion	Hydroxyl palmitoyl sphinganines—ceramide precursor, L-arginine, sodium PCA, allantoin and panthenol, glycerin, pentylene glycol, sorbitol, cyclopentasiloxane and dimethiconol, cetyl alcohol, sunflower seed oil, caprylyl glycol
Cetaphil bar (moisturising soap)	Syndet base 98.5%, shea blend 10%, perfume 0.5%
Sebamed moisturizing cream for sensitive skin pH 5.5	Aqua, petrolatum, myreth-3 myristate, glycerin, cetearyl alcohol, tocopheryl acetate, ceteareth-20, dimethicone, sodium PCA, sodium citrate, sodium carbomer, perfume, benzyl alcohol, phenoxyethanol
Sebamed baby lotion	
Sebamed baby cream extra soft	42% lipids, panthenol
Sebamed clear face care gel for acne prone skin Free from oils and emulsifiers	Aqua, *Aloe barbadensis* leaf juice, propylene glycol, glycerin, sorbitol, panthenol, sodium hyaluronate, allantoin, sodium carbomer, sodium citrate, phenoxyethanol
Sebamed anti dry hydrating body lotion	Phytosterols, vitamin E, phytopeptides, shea butter
Sebamed cleansing bar For normal to oily skin, soap free	Disodium lauryl sulfosuccinate, *Triticum vulgare* starch, palmitic acid, stearic acid, glyceryl stearate, cetearyl alcohol, talc, sodium lactate, cera alba, aqua, lecithin, sodium lauryl sarcosinate, cocamidopropyl betaine, panthenol, inulin, sodium cocoyl glutamate, tocopheryl acetate, glycerin, magnesium aspartate, alanine, lysine, leucine, benzophenone-4, perfume, CI 47005, CI 61570, CI 77891

Continued

Continued

Name of the product	Ingredients
Acrofy	Purified water, glycerin, propylene glycol, niacinamide, aqua-butylene glycol-PEG-60 almond glycerides-caprylyl glycol-glycerin-carbomer-nordihydroguaiaretic acid-oleanolic acid, *Imperata cylindrica*-aqua-glycerin-PEG 8-carbomer, polyamide 5, shea butter, glyceryl stearate, PEG 100 stearate, cetyl alcohol, cyclomethicone and dimethicone copolyol, ethylhexyl palmitate-sorbitan oleate-sorbitan laurate-myristyl phosphor-malate, sodium acrylates copolymer lecithin, sodium gluconate and lactate derivative, stearyl alcohol, sorbitan monostearate, citric acid, propyl paraben, BHT, disodium edentate, methyl paraben, ascorbyl palmitate
LacSoft	Ammonium lactate 12% w/w
Cutimax cream	White liquid paraffin 13.2%, LLP 10.2%, in glycerin base
LacSoft C gel	Clobetasol propionate 0.05%, ammonium lactate 12%
Allograce cream	Aloe vera extract 10%, wheat germ oil (natural vitamin E) 0.6%, honey extract 1%, tea tree oil 0.1%
Aveeno DML lotion Daily moisturizing lotion	Aqua, glycerin, distearyldimonium chloride, petrolatum, isopropyl palmitate, cetyl alcohol, dimethicone, *Avena sativa* (oat) kernel flour, benzyl alcohol, sodium chloride
Aveeno SRL lotion Skin relief moisturizing lotion	Aqua, glycerin, distearyldimonium chloride, petrolatum, isopropyl palmitate, cetyl alcohol, dimethicone, *Avena sativa* (oat) kernel flour, *A. sativa* (oat) kernel oil, benzyl alcohol, *Butyrospermum parkii* (shea butter) extract, Steareth-20, *A. sativa* (oat) kernel extract, sodium chloride
Physiogel cream	Ceramide, triglycerides, glycerin, squalane, hydrogenated lecithin
Physiogel lotion	Ceramide, triglycerides, glycerin, squalane, hydrogenated lecithin
Physiogel AI cream	Palmitamide MEA, ceramide, triglycerides, glycerin, squalane, hydrogenated lecithin
Physiogel AI lotion	Palmitamide MEA, ceramide, triglycerides, glycerin, squalane, hydrogenated lecithin
Oilatum cream	Light liquid paraffin, white soft paraffin
Oilatum lotion	Light liquid paraffin, white soft paraffin, providone K29, shea butter, glycerin
Oilatum emollient	Light liquid paraffin-63.4% w/w, Isopropyl plamitate, Isopropyl alcohol
Oilatum bar	Mineral oil, sodium palmate, glycerin
Emoderm cream	White soft paraffin

LLP, light liquid paraffin; BHT, butylated hydroxytoluene; BHA, butylated hydroxyanisole; PEG, polyethylene glycol; DMDM, 1,3-dimethylol-5,5-dimethylhydantoin; EDTA, ethylenediaminetetraacetic acid; MBBT, methylene bis-benzotriazolyl tetramethylbutylphenol; PCA, pyrrolidone carboxylic acid; MEA, monoethanolamine.

Printed by Libri Plureos GmbH in Hamburg, Germany